The Biology of Aging: What Happens at the Cellular and Molecular Levels?

A very short introduction from
The HealthSpan Institute

Contents

Preface

Chapter 1: Introduction to Aging

Chapter 2: The Cellular Landscape

Chapter 3: Telomeres and Telomerase

Chapter 4: Mitochondrial Dynamics

Chapter 5: DNA Damage and Repair

Chapter 6: Cellular Senescence

Chapter 7: Autophagy and Protein Homeostasis

Chapter 8: The Role of Epigenetics in Aging

Chapter 9: Inflammation and Aging

Chapter 10: Intercellular Communication and the Aging Microenvironment

Chapter 11: Hallmarks of Aging

Chapter 12: Interventions and the Future of Age Biology

Preface

Why Understanding the Biology of Aging is Essential

Aging is an inevitable process that every living organism undergoes, from the tiniest microbe to the largest mammals. As the years pass, human beings, in particular, experience a myriad of physiological, cognitive, and aesthetic changes. With an aging global population, understanding the biology of aging has never been more critical. Here are several compelling reasons why delving into the cellular and molecular intricacies of aging is essential.

1. **Improving Quality of Life:** As individuals grow older, they often face numerous health challenges, from reduced cognitive abilities to physical frailty. A deep understanding of the biology of aging can offer insights into how to counteract or delay these debilitating changes. By understanding the root causes of age-related decline at the cellular and molecular levels, scientists can potentially develop interventions that enhance the healthspan of individuals, ensuring that our later years are not just longer, but also healthier and more vibrant.

2. **Addressing Age-related Diseases:** Many diseases, including Alzheimer's, Parkinson's, cardiovascular diseases, and certain cancers, have a higher incidence in older populations. Grasping the biology of aging can lead to a more profound understanding of why these diseases occur more frequently as we age. This knowledge can, in turn, pave the way for better preventive strategies, more effective treatments, and even potential cures.

3. **Economic Implications:** With the rise in life expectancy in many parts of the world, there's an increasing proportion of elderly individuals in the global population. This demographic shift has profound economic implications. Older populations often require more medical care, leading to increased healthcare costs. By understanding and potentially mitigating the adverse effects of aging, societies can reduce healthcare burdens and ensure

that older individuals can remain economically active for longer, benefiting economies at large.

4. **Advancing Fundamental Science:** Aging is a complex process influenced by a plethora of genetic, environmental, and lifestyle factors. Studying aging can help unravel fundamental biological mysteries. For instance, why do some organisms age faster than others? How do certain animals, like the Greenland shark or the bowhead whale, live for hundreds of years? Delving into these questions can lead to profound discoveries about life, evolution, and the very nature of existence.

5. **Ethical Considerations:** The quest for longevity, if not immortality, has been a part of human lore and desire for millennia. As we inch closer to realizing some of these aspirations through scientific advancements, understanding the biology of aging becomes paramount to making informed ethical decisions. Should we pursue treatments that extend life indefinitely? What are the societal implications of a significantly increased lifespan? A foundational knowledge of the aging process ensures that such discussions are grounded in fact rather than fiction.

6. **Shaping Healthcare Policies:** An understanding of the biology of aging will influence public health recommendations and policies. For instance, if certain molecular pathways are found to play pivotal roles in aging, public health campaigns might emphasize lifestyle choices that positively influence these pathways. Similarly, healthcare systems can be better designed to address the unique needs of an aging population.

In conclusion, the biology of aging is not just a topic of academic interest; it has profound implications for individuals and societies. As poet Dylan Thomas wrote, "Do not go gentle into that good night," a sentiment that resonates with many who hope to age with vigor and grace. By deepening our understanding of the aging process, we equip ourselves with the knowledge to make that hope a tangible reality. Aging, in all its complexity, offers a window into the intricacies of life, and understanding it holds the promise of better health, robust economies, and more informed ethical choices for the future.

Scope and Structure of the Book

The Scope

"The Biology of Aging: What Happens at the Cellular and Molecular Levels?" aims to provide a comprehensive exploration into the intricate processes that drive aging at the most fundamental levels. Our journey will traverse the microscopic realm, delving deep into cells and molecules, uncovering the myriad changes that accompany the passage of time.

Our examination isn't just academic. By understanding these processes, we can shed light on age-related diseases, the challenges of an aging population, and potential interventions that might one day slow or even reverse aspects of the aging process. This book is designed to be a bridge between complex scientific concepts and an audience eager for knowledge, whether they are students, professionals, or anyone curious about the ticking biological clock within us all.

The Structure:

The book is structured to provide a logical progression from foundational concepts to more advanced topics, ensuring readers develop a step-by-step understanding of the biology of aging.

Foundational Chapters: The initial sections introduce the reader to the basics of cellular biology, offering context for the subsequent, more detailed discussions about aging. These chapters will lay the groundwork, ensuring all readers, regardless of their background, can grasp the complexities of the topics that follow.

Core Content: The heart of the book delves into specific mechanisms and hallmarks of aging, from telomeres and their influence on cellular senescence to the role of mitochondria, DNA damage, and repair mechanisms. Each chapter is devoted to a particular aspect or pathway, providing in-depth exploration supplemented with diagrams, case studies, and the latest research findings.

Integrative Insights: As we move deeper into the book, the focus will shift from individual mechanisms to how these processes interplay and influence one another, providing a holistic view of the aging process.

Future Prospects: The final chapters are forward-looking, discussing potential interventions, cutting-edge research, and the ethical and societal implications of extending human lifespan. These chapters will highlight where the field is heading and the challenges and opportunities that lie ahead.

Throughout the book, sidebars will offer additional information on related topics, historical perspectives, and current research breakthroughs. A glossary at the end will ensure readers have a quick reference for any terms or concepts they wish to revisit.

In essence, "The Biology of Aging: What Happens at the Cellular and Molecular Levels?" is structured to be both a guide and a journey, taking readers from the basics to the frontiers of aging research, demystifying complex processes and highlighting the profound impact of time on our very cells and molecules.

Chapter 1: Introduction to Aging

Defining Aging: Biological vs. Chronological Age

Aging, a universal process, is integral to the tapestry of life. As the years accumulate, changes manifest in our bodies, minds, and even our very cells. But how we define and measure aging can vary significantly. The most common distinction is between chronological age, the literal time we've existed, and biological age, the physical and functional state of our bodies. Understanding the differences between these two concepts is crucial for both scientific research and our perception of health and longevity.

Chronological Age

Chronological age is the most straightforward measure of aging; it represents the time that has passed since our birth. Celebrated through annual birthdays, this metric is used universally to determine life stages, from childhood and adolescence to adulthood and old age. Chronological age provides a handy reference point for societal norms and expectations, influencing decisions about education, work, retirement, and more.

However, while chronological age is consistent (a year is a year for everyone), its relationship to health, vitality, and functionality can vary immensely among individuals. Two people, both 60 years old, might have dramatically different physical abilities, cognitive functions, and health profiles. This discrepancy brings us to the concept of biological age.

Biological Age

Biological age paints a more intricate picture of aging, reflecting the physiological and functional state of an organism. It captures the disparities mentioned above and is shaped by a combination of genetics, lifestyle, environmental factors, and random biological events. While chronological age marches forward uniformly, biological age can vary, influenced by how our bodies respond to both internal and external stresses.

Several markers can be used to assess biological age:

- **Cellular markers:** These include telomere length (the protective caps on the ends of our chromosomes that tend to shorten as we age), cellular senescence (when cells lose their ability to divide and function), and mitochondrial function.
- **Molecular markers:** Biomarkers in the blood, like inflammatory molecules or DNA methylation patterns, can provide insights into our biological age.
- **Functional markers:** These encompass a range of physiological attributes, from cardiovascular and lung function to cognitive assessments and muscle strength.

Using a combination of these markers, researchers have developed various models to estimate biological age. Interestingly, studies have shown that one's biological age might be a better predictor of health, disease onset, and mortality than chronological age.

Implications of the Distinction

The separation between biological and chronological age has significant implications for both individuals and societies. On an individual level, understanding that our choices and environments can influence our biological age provides an empowering perspective. It suggests that through lifestyle modifications, like a balanced diet, regular exercise, stress management, and avoiding toxins, we might positively influence our biological aging process, potentially leading to a healthier and longer life.

From a societal standpoint, as the global population grows older, there's a heightened emphasis on "healthy aging." With the knowledge that chronological age doesn't necessarily equate to health or disease status, healthcare systems can focus on interventions that target biological aging, offering more personalized and effective treatments.

Conclusion

In essence, while chronological age offers a consistent metric of time, it's the biological age that provides deeper insights into our state of health and the aging process. By defining and differentiating these two aspects of age, we can better understand the intricacies of aging, paving the way for scientific advancements and personal choices that can lead to longer, healthier lives.

Theories of Aging: Overview and Historical Perspectives

Aging, a universal phenomenon observed across various species, has fascinated scientists, philosophers, and thinkers for centuries. The desire to understand why organisms grow old and the underlying mechanisms of this process has led to the proposal of multiple theories. While no single theory exclusively explains the intricacies of aging, collectively they offer a rich tapestry of insights that have evolved over time.

Historical Perspectives on Aging

Historically, ancient civilizations often linked aging to the whims of gods, natural cycles, or cosmic events. For instance, the Greeks believed in the Three Fates, who determined the lifespan of every individual: one spun the thread of life, the other measured it, and the third cut it. Chinese philosophy emphasized the balance of yin and yang, with imbalances leading to aging and disease.

As scientific inquiry advanced, especially during the Renaissance, there was a shift towards seeking natural and biological explanations for aging. This transition set the stage for the myriad of aging theories that we have today.

Stochastic Theories

These theories suggest that aging results from accumulated random damages at the cellular and molecular levels.

1. **Wear and Tear Theory:** One of the earliest scientific theories, it posits that like machines, bodies wear out from repeated use. This wear and tear at the cellular level leads to aging and eventually death. However, this theory alone doesn't explain why organisms have varying lifespans or why certain repairs can extend life.

2. **Free Radical Theory:** Proposed in the 1950s by Denham Harman, this theory suggests that reactive oxygen species (ROS), a byproduct of metabolic processes, can cause cellular damage, particularly to DNA, proteins, and lipids. Over time, this cumulative damage contributes to aging and age-related diseases.

Programmatic Theories

These theories suggest that aging is predetermined and programmed into the very genes and biological processes of organisms.

1. **Genetic Program Theory:** This theory proposes that aging is directed by specific genes that control developmental processes. As organisms reach maturity and reproduction, these genes, having fulfilled their primary evolutionary purpose, might lead to aging as a side effect.

2. **Telomere Shortening:** Telomeres, protective sequences at the end of chromosomes, shorten as cells divide. When they become critically short, cells enter a state of senescence or programmed cell death. This process is considered a form of biological clock, leading to aging and eventual death.

Integrated Theories

Recent advances suggest that aging might be a combination of stochastic and programmatic factors.

1. **Damage and Repair Mechanism:** This approach acknowledges that while stochastic events cause damage, organisms possess repair mechanisms. Aging results when the rate of damage exceeds repair capabilities.

2. **Evolutionary Theories:** Aging might be a byproduct of natural selection. Organisms are optimized for reproduction and survival until they reproduce. Beyond this reproductive window, the evolutionary pressures are weak, allowing aging and age-related diseases to manifest.

Conclusion

From the musings of ancient civilizations to contemporary genetic research, our understanding of aging has evolved significantly. The variety of theories proposed throughout history reflects the complexity of the aging process itself. While each theory offers a unique lens through which to view aging, it's likely that the true nature of aging integrates elements from multiple theories.

As we continue to uncover the mysteries of biology and delve deeper into the molecular intricacies of life, our perspectives on aging will continue to evolve, reshaping the ways in which we approach longevity, health, and the very essence of life itself.

Why Do Organisms Age?

One of the most profound and universal questions in biology pertains to the nature of aging: Why do organisms age? Why isn't immortality, or at least an indefinitely prolonged youth, the standard for biological entities? The aging phenomenon, observed across a vast spectrum of species, from microscopic organisms to plants and animals, offers fascinating insights into the intricacies of life.

Cellular Mechanisms

At the cellular level, numerous processes contribute to aging.

1. **DNA Damage:** Over time, an organism's DNA accumulates damage from various sources, including environmental factors like radiation and internal factors such as replication errors. While cells have repair mechanisms, they aren't foolproof. Accumulated DNA damage can lead to cell malfunction or cell death.

2. **Telomere Shortening:** Each time a cell divides, the telomeres at the end of its chromosomes shorten. After multiple divisions, the telomeres become critically short, preventing further divisions and leading to cell senescence or apoptosis.

3. **Mitochondrial Dysfunction:** Mitochondria, the powerhouses of cells, produce energy but also reactive oxygen species (ROS) as a byproduct. Over time, the damage from ROS, combined with other factors, can lead to reduced mitochondrial efficiency, affecting cellular function.

Evolutionary Theories

Aging, surprisingly, can be contextualized within the framework of evolution.

1. **Disposable Soma Theory:** This theory suggests a trade-off between reproduction and maintenance. Energy is a finite resource. Organisms prioritize energy towards reproduction, sometimes at the expense of maintenance and repair. Over time, this neglect manifests as aging.

2. **Antagonistic Pleiotropy:** Proposed by George Williams in 1957, this theory posits that some genes which are beneficial in youth (enhancing fertility or survival) might have detrimental effects in later life. Since natural selection acts most strongly on traits expressed before reproduction, genes that are beneficial early on but harmful later might still be favored and passed on.

Life History and Ecological Factors:

An organism's environment and life strategy also play roles in aging.

1. **Predation and External Risks:** In environments with high predation or external risks, there's a higher premium on early reproduction. Organisms might evolve to mature and reproduce quickly, even if it means a shorter overall lifespan.

2. **Reproductive Strategies:** Some organisms, like Pacific salmon, exhibit "semelparity," where they reproduce once and then die.

Others, like humans, have "iteroparous" life histories, reproducing multiple times and living beyond reproductive age. These strategies can influence aging patterns.

Biochemical and Metabolic Processes:

1. **Protein Aggregation:** Over time, misfolded proteins can accumulate in cells, leading to reduced cellular function and diseases like Alzheimer's.

2. **Glycation:** Sugars can react with proteins, lipids, or nucleic acids, leading to advanced glycation end products (AGEs). AGEs can affect cellular function and are linked to various age-related diseases.

3. **Hormonal Changes:** Hormones regulate various physiological processes. As organisms age, hormonal levels and responses can change, affecting everything from metabolism to immune function.

Conclusion:

The question of why organisms age remains one of the most captivating puzzles in biology. While there isn't a singular answer, the amalgamation of cellular, evolutionary, ecological, and biochemical factors provides a multifaceted explanation. Aging, it seems, is the complex interplay of genetics, environment, energy trade-offs, and the inevitable wear and tear of biological processes. Understanding this interplay not only offers insights into the nature of life and evolution but also holds the promise of interventions that can enhance health and longevity.

Chapter 2: The Cellular Landscape

Basics of Cellular Biology

Cellular biology, often referred to as cell biology, delves into the microscopic world of cells, the fundamental units of life. From single-celled bacteria to the myriad cells comprising complex multicellular organisms like humans, cellular biology offers insights into the structure, function, and intricate processes that sustain life.

Cell Theory

Modern cellular biology is rooted in the cell theory, which posits:

1. All living organisms are composed of one or more cells.

2. The cell is the basic unit of structure and organization in organisms.

3. All cells arise from pre-existing cells.

Basic Cell Structure

Cells, though diverse in function and appearance, share some common structural elements:

1. **Cell Membrane:** This semi-permeable barrier surrounds the cell, regulating the entry and exit of substances. It's primarily composed of a phospholipid bilayer, interspersed with proteins.

2. **Cytoplasm:** The jelly-like substance within the cell membrane, excluding the nucleus, contains various organelles, each with a specific function.

3. **Nucleus:** Found in eukaryotic cells, the nucleus houses the cell's genetic material, DNA. It's enveloped by the nuclear membrane and regulates gene expression.

4. **Mitochondria:** Often termed the "powerhouse" of the cell, mitochondria are responsible for producing adenosine triphosphate (ATP), the cell's energy currency, through a process called cellular respiration.

5. **Endoplasmic Reticulum (ER):** This membranous network is involved in protein synthesis (rough ER) and lipid metabolism (smooth ER).

6. **Golgi Apparatus:** It modifies, sorts, and packages proteins and lipids for transport to their designated locations.

7. **Lysosomes:** Containing digestive enzymes, lysosomes break down waste materials and cellular debris.

8. **Ribosomes:** These are the protein factories of the cell, synthesizing proteins based on the instructions from DNA.

Types of Cells

There are two primary cell types based on complexity and the presence or absence of specific structures:

1. **Prokaryotic Cells:** These are simpler and smaller cells without a defined nucleus. Their genetic material is found in a region called the nucleoid. Bacteria are classic examples of prokaryotes.

2. **Eukaryotic Cells:** More complex than their prokaryotic counterparts, eukaryotic cells contain a nucleus and various other organelles. Plants, animals, fungi, and protists are all composed of eukaryotic cells.

Cellular Processes

Cells are hubs of activity, orchestrating a myriad of processes to maintain homeostasis and ensure survival:

1. **Cell Division:** Cells reproduce through division. Prokaryotes typically utilize binary fission, while eukaryotes undergo mitosis (for growth and repair) or meiosis (for sexual reproduction).

2. **Metabolism:** Cells conduct a series of chemical reactions to produce energy, build cellular structures, and dispose of waste. This includes pathways like glycolysis, the Krebs cycle, and oxidative phosphorylation.

3. **Protein Synthesis:** Using instructions encoded in DNA, cells synthesize proteins, which play vital roles, from acting as enzymes to providing structural support.

4. **Cell Signaling:** Cells communicate using signaling molecules, allowing them to respond to changes in their environment or coordinate activities with other cells.

Conclusion:

Cells are marvels of biological engineering. Their intricate structures and processes underpin the complexity of life itself. From the simple division of bacterial cells to the sophisticated signaling networks in human cells, cellular biology offers a window into the dynamic, ever-evolving world of life at its most fundamental level. As we delve deeper into the topic of aging, understanding these basics will serve as a foundation, illuminating the cellular and molecular changes that accompany the passage of time.

Cell Cycle, Differentiation, and the Significance of Stem Cells

As the study of cellular biology advances, it becomes evident that cells, while being life's foundational units, are far from static entities. They undergo cycles of division, can specialize into diverse forms, and possess the unique ability to regenerate and repair tissues. This section delves into the cell cycle, the process of differentiation, and the unparalleled significance of stem cells.

Cell Cycle

The cell cycle is a series of events that lead to cell growth and division into two daughter cells. It is typically divided into two main phases:

1. **Interphase:** This is the phase where the cell grows and prepares for division. It consists of:

   - **G1 phase (Gap 1):** Cellular content, excluding chromosomes, is duplicated.
   - **S phase (Synthesis):** DNA is replicated.
   - **G2 phase (Gap 2):** Further growth occurs, and the cell prepares for division.

2. **Mitotic (M) Phase:** The cell divides during this phase, which includes:

   - **Mitosis:** The nucleus divides into two nuclei, each with identical DNA.
   - **Cytokinesis:** The cytoplasm divides, resulting in two distinct daughter cells.

Differentiation

Every multicellular organism starts as a single fertilized egg cell, or zygote. As this cell divides, its descendants undergo a process of differentiation, becoming specialized in their functions and forms. This specialization is crucial for the development of diverse tissues and organs.

Differentiation is regulated by a variety of internal and external cues, including gene expression, hormones, and cell-to-cell interactions. As cells differentiate, they gradually lose their ability to become any cell type, becoming committed to a particular lineage.

Stem Cells and Their Significance

At the heart of differentiation and the ability to generate diverse cell types are stem cells. These are unique cells with two critical properties:

1. **Self-Renewal:** They can divide and produce identical daughter stem cells.

2. **Differentiation Potential:** They can give rise to specialized cell types.

There are various types of stem cells, each with different capabilities:

1. **Totipotent Stem Cells:** These can give rise to all cell types, including the cells that make up the placenta. The fertilized egg and the cells it divides into in the earliest stages of embryonic development are totipotent.

2. **Pluripotent Stem Cells:** These can give rise to all cell types of the body but not the placenta. Embryonic stem cells, derived from early-stage embryos, are pluripotent.

3. **Multipotent Stem Cells:** These can produce cells of a particular lineage. Hematopoietic stem cells, for instance, can give rise to various types of blood cells but not to other cell types.

4. **Induced Pluripotent Stem Cells (iPSCs):** Scientists have discovered ways to reprogram specialized adult cells to assume a stem cell-like state, termed as iPSCs. These cells hold promise for regenerative medicine without the ethical concerns tied to embryonic stem cells.

Stem cells play vital roles throughout an organism's life:

- **Development:** Stem cells help in forming the various tissues and organs during embryonic and early postnatal life.
- **Repair and Regeneration:** In many tissues, like the skin and blood, stem cells replace worn-out or damaged cells.
- **Medical Potential:** Because of their regenerative capabilities, stem cells hold tremendous promise for treating diseases, from neurodegenerative conditions to heart diseases.

Conclusion

The intricate dance of the cell cycle and differentiation underpins the development, growth, and repair mechanisms of all multicellular organisms. Stem cells, with their unique properties, stand at the forefront of this biological marvel, heralding possibilities that could redefine medical science. As we explore aging at the cellular level, understanding these processes becomes paramount, offering clues into how cells change over time and how they might be harnessed to promote health and longevity.

How Cells Communicate: Signaling Pathways and Their Relevance to Aging

Within the vast multicellular tapestry of organisms, individual cells are not isolated entities. Instead, they engage in continuous, dynamic dialogues with their neighbors, orchestrating a harmonious interplay of functions. This communication is pivotal for maintaining homeostasis, coordinating growth, and responding to external stimuli. However, as organisms age, some of these signaling pathways may falter or change, contributing to the aging process and age-related diseases. Here, we delve into the fundamentals of cellular communication and its significance in aging.

The Basics of Cell Signaling

Cellular communication hinges on signaling molecules and receptors. The process can be summarized in a few key steps:

1. **Signal Generation:** A cell (sender) produces a signaling molecule, often in response to an internal or external change.

2. **Release and Transport:** The signaling molecule is released and travels to its target, either through diffusion (in short distances) or through the bloodstream (for distant targets).

3. **Reception:** The target cell (receiver) has specific receptors that can recognize and bind to the signaling molecule.

4. **Signal Transduction:** Upon binding, the receptor undergoes a change, initiating a cascade of intracellular events that translate the external signal into a functional response.

5. **Response:** The target cell alters its behavior or function in response to the received signal.

Types of Cell Signaling

1. **Autocrine Signaling:** Cells send signals to themselves. A cell produces signaling molecules that bind to its own receptors, influencing its behavior.

2. **Paracrine Signaling:** Signals are sent to nearby cells. Examples include neurotransmitters and growth factors.

3. **Endocrine Signaling:** Signals are sent over long distances, usually through the bloodstream. Hormones, like insulin or estrogen, are typical examples.

4. **Juxtacrine Signaling:** Direct cell-to-cell contact, where signaling molecules remain bound to the cell surface of the signaling cell and influence adjacent cells.

Relevance to Aging

Cell signaling pathways play pivotal roles in the aging process and in age-related diseases. Here's how:

1. **Regulation of Growth and Repair:** Signaling molecules like growth factors regulate cell growth, division, and repair. As organisms age, there can be changes in the levels or activity of these molecules, affecting tissue maintenance and function.

2. **Stress Response:** Cells have signaling pathways, such as the MAPK pathway, that respond to stressors like oxidative damage. Aging might attenuate the efficacy of these pathways, making cells more vulnerable to damage.

3. **Inflammation:** Chronic, low-grade inflammation, termed "inflammaging," is a hallmark of aging. Dysregulated signaling, involving molecules like cytokines, can lead to persistent inflammation, contributing to age-related disorders.

4. **Metabolic Signaling:** Aging affects metabolic pathways, including those regulated by molecules like insulin and mTOR. Alterations in these pathways can influence lifespan and age-associated diseases.

5. **Stem Cell Signaling:** As organisms age, signaling pathways in stem cells can change, affecting their ability to regenerate tissues.

Conclusion

The intricate web of cell signaling ensures seamless communication, allowing cells to adapt, grow, and function optimally. However, as the sands of time shift, these pathways may undergo alterations, some subtle and others more pronounced. Understanding these changes, and how they intertwine with the aging process, can offer insights into potential interventions, from lifestyle adjustments to therapeutic strategies. By decoding the symphony of cellular communication and its variations over time, we move a step closer to unraveling the mysteries of aging and ensuring a healthier, more graceful dance with time.

Chapter 3: Telomeres and Telomerase

Introduction to Telomeres: Their Role and Structure

The vast intricacies of cellular biology often lead to comparisons with intricate machinery. And like a well-made machine, each part, no matter how tiny, has a specific and critical function. Among these numerous components are telomeres, which can be likened to the protective caps on shoelaces. Their role, primarily associated with cellular aging and genomic stability, is pivotal, and any disruption to their function has far-reaching implications for health and longevity. In this section, we delve into the fundamental nature of telomeres, their role, and their intricate structure.

What are Telomeres?

Telomeres are repetitive sequences of non-coding DNA located at the ends of chromosomes. Their primary purpose is to protect the vital genetic information encoded within our DNA. As cells divide, the DNA replication process cannot fully replicate the very ends of chromosomes, which means that with each cell division, the telomeres shorten slightly. Hence, telomeres serve as buffers, ensuring that the shortening doesn't immediately affect the essential coding regions of our DNA.

The Role of Telomeres

1. **Protection of Genetic Information:** The primary function of telomeres is to safeguard the ends of chromosomes from deterioration or from fusion with neighboring chromosomes. They achieve this by preventing the cellular machinery from misidentifying the chromosome ends as broken DNA, which, if left unchecked, could lead to errors in DNA repair mechanisms.

2. **Cellular Aging Indicator:** Telomere length serves as a kind of biological clock for cells. With each cell division, telomeres shorten, and after a certain number of divisions, they reach a critical length. Once this occurs, cells enter a state of senescence or programmed cell death (apoptosis). This mechanism prevents the propagation of errors in cell replication, which might lead to malignancies or other cellular dysfunctions.

3. **Role in Cancer:** Some cells, notably cancer cells, can activate an enzyme called telomerase that rebuilds telomeres, allowing the cells to divide indefinitely. This capacity for unlimited division is a hallmark of many types of cancer.

4. **Genomic Stability:** By preventing chromosome fusion and maintaining chromosome integrity, telomeres play a pivotal role in ensuring that the genome remains stable and that genetic information is passed accurately during cell division.

Structure of Telomeres

At a molecular level, telomeres have a specific structure that distinguishes them from other DNA sequences:

1. **DNA Sequence:** The exact sequence of telomeres can vary across species, but in humans, it is typically composed of thousands of repeats of the sequence TTAGGG.

2. **Strand Overhang:** The telomeric DNA has a double-stranded region and a single-stranded overhang, with the latter being rich in the base Guanine. This overhang can fold back and invade the double-stranded region, forming a protective structure called a T-loop.

3. **Telomere-binding Proteins:** Telomeres aren't just bare sequences of DNA; they are associated with a range of specialized proteins that ensure their stability and proper function. These proteins, collectively referred to as the shelterin complex, recognize and bind to the telomeric sequences, protecting them and assisting in the formation of the T-loop structure.

Conclusion

Telomeres, despite being a small segment at the end of chromosomes, play an outsized role in cellular health, aging, and genomic stability. Their dynamic nature, shortening with each cell division and occasionally being rebuilt, connects them directly to the biological processes that define the life of a cell. As we delve deeper into the complexities of aging, understanding telomeres and their interplay with other cellular components becomes crucial. Their potential as therapeutic targets, especially in age-related diseases, is an exciting frontier in modern biology and medicine.

Telomere Shortening and Cellular Senescence

In the ceaseless dance of life, cells constantly grow, divide, and eventually, meet their end. This cycle, central to the vitality of all multicellular organisms, is inextricably linked with the phenomenon of telomere shortening and its eventual outcome: cellular senescence. These processes are not merely academic curiosities; they bear profound implications for aging, tissue regeneration, and a plethora of age-related diseases.

The Mechanics of Telomere Shortening:

At the heart of cellular replication lies the DNA replication process. As cells prepare to divide, enzymes work diligently to replicate the DNA so that each daughter cell inherits an identical set. But there's a snag. Due to the mechanics of DNA replication, the replication machinery cannot fully replicate the extreme ends of linear DNA. With each replication cycle, a small portion of the telomere is lost, leading to progressive shortening.

To visualize this, consider a photocopier that, no matter how advanced, always misses the last line of a page. If you were to repeatedly copy the last copy produced, over time, more and more of the original content would be lost. Telomeres act as expendable buffers, similar to those bottom lines, ensuring that the main content – the vital genetic information – remains intact for as many replications as possible.

Enter Cellular Senescence

So, what happens when telomeres reach a critically short length? Cells enter a state known as senescence. Cellular senescence is a state of irreversible growth arrest, meaning the cell no longer divides. But these senescent cells are not dormant; they often exhibit changes in metabolism, function, and morphology. Moreover, they can secrete pro-inflammatory molecules, contributing to what is known as the senescence-associated secretory phenotype (SASP).

Three primary factors highlight the significance of cellular senescence:

1. **Tumor Suppression:** At first glance, cellular senescence seems counterproductive. Why have a mechanism that curtails the lifespan of a cell? The answer lies in cancer prevention. By halting the growth of cells with dangerously short telomeres, senescence prevents genomic instability – a precursor to cancer.

2. **Tissue Aging:** While senescence has protective roles, an accumulation of senescent cells in tissues over time can promote aging. The SASP can induce inflammation and impede tissue repair, both of which contribute to aging and age-related pathologies.

3. **Implications for Regenerative Medicine:** Stem cells, which replenish tissues, also experience telomere shortening and senescence. As we age, the diminished capacity of stem cells to repair and regenerate tissue can lead to various degenerative diseases.

Telomerase: A Counter to Shortening

Nature, in its foresight, does have a mechanism to counter telomere shortening: the enzyme telomerase. Telomerase can add telomeric repeats to the ends of chromosomes, effectively rebuilding the telomere. However, its activity is generally suppressed in most somatic cells, presumably as a defense against uncontrolled cell growth. In stem cells and certain other cells, telomerase activity is maintained, granting them a longer replicative lifespan.

Conclusion

The relationship between telomere shortening and cellular senescence epitomizes the delicate balance between protective and degenerative mechanisms in biology. While telomere shortening serves as a checkpoint against unchecked cell proliferation, the resultant cellular senescence, especially when accumulated, plays a role in tissue aging and dysfunction. The study of these processes, therefore, holds promise not just for understanding aging but also for devising interventions that might one day mitigate age-associated decline and diseases.

Telomerase and Its Therapeutic Potential in Aging

In the vast panorama of cellular biology, telomerase stands as a beacon of intrigue and potential. This enzyme, tasked with the duty of maintaining the protective caps of chromosomes, the telomeres, has sparked significant interest in the realms of aging research and therapy. But why is there such fervor around telomerase, and how might it be harnessed therapeutically to address age-related challenges?

Telomerase: A Primer

Telomerase is a ribonucleoprotein enzyme complex responsible for elongating telomeres, the DNA-protein structures at the ends of chromosomes. As cells divide, telomeres naturally shorten due to the limitations of the DNA replication process. Once telomeres reach a critically short length, cells enter a state of senescence, halting further division. Telomerase counteracts this by adding telomeric DNA sequences, ensuring that cells can continue to divide and remain functional.

In humans, high telomerase activity is primarily found in stem cells, germ cells, and certain white blood cells. Its activity is notably suppressed in most somatic cells, likely as a protective mechanism against uncontrolled cell proliferation and cancer.

30

Therapeutic Potential in Aging:

1. **Extending Cellular Lifespan:** Given its role in maintaining telomere length, telomerase has the potential to extend the replicative lifespan of cells. By delaying cellular senescence, tissues
   could theoretically regenerate and function efficiently for more
   extended periods.

2. **Counteracting Age-Related Diseases:** A significant portion of
   age-related diseases, such as certain degenerative disorders and
   tissue dysfunctions, can be traced back to cellular senescence
   and the resulting loss of tissue regenerative capacity. By upregu-
   lating telomerase activity, it might be possible to mitigate some
   of these conditions.

3. **Enhancing Stem Cell Function:** Stem cells serve as the regenerative powerhouses of tissues, replenishing cells and maintaining
   tissue function. However, with age, their regenerative potential
   wanes, in part due to telomere shortening. Elevating telomerase
   activity in stem cells might rejuvenate their regenerative prowess.

Challenges and Considerations

Harnessing telomerase for therapeutic purposes is not without challenges:

1. **Cancer Risk:** The most pressing concern is the potential for uncontrolled cell growth. Telomerase is active in many cancer cells,
   allowing them to bypass senescence and proliferate indefinitely.
   Therapeutically increasing telomerase activity could inadvertent-
   ly heighten the risk of cancer.

2. **Delivery Mechanisms:** Efficiently delivering telomerase or its
   activating agents to target cells in a controlled manner remains a
   challenge. While viral vectors are commonly used in gene therapy, they come with their own set of risks and limitations.

3. **Potential for Aging Reversal vs. Aging Delay:** While telomerase
   could potentially delay aging by extending the functional lifespan of cells, whether it can reverse existing cellular and tissue
   damage remains a subject of intense research.

Current Research and Future Directions

Several studies have delved into the therapeutic potential of telomerase. Some have explored small molecules that can activate telomerase,
while others have looked into gene therapies that introduce telomerase into cells. Animal models, particularly mice with engineered
telomerase expression, have shown promising results in terms of
healthspan extension and delayed aging.

Conclusion

Telomerase, with its intimate connection to cellular aging, offers a tantalizing avenue for therapeutic interventions in aging and age-related
diseases. While the potential benefits are profound, the challenges are
equally significant. As researchers continue to unravel the complexities
of telomerase regulation and function, the dream of harnessing its
powers for human health and longevity draws ever closer. The journey
promises not only to expand our understanding of cellular aging but
also to redefine the boundaries of therapeutic possibilities.

Chapter 4: Mitochondrial Dynamics

The Powerhouse of the Cell: Basics of Mitochondria

In the intricate metropolis of the cell, the mitochondria stand out as essential energy hubs, frequently hailed as the "powerhouses" of the cell. Beyond just energy production, their multifaceted roles encompass various cellular processes, including calcium signaling, apoptosis, and even the synthesis of certain biomolecules. Delving into the basics of mitochondria provides a foundation for understanding cellular metabolism, vitality, and the deeper intricacies of aging and disease.

Origin and Structure of Mitochondria

The origins of mitochondria are a tale of symbiosis. Evolutionary evidence suggests that they originated from a free-living bacterium that was engulfed by an ancestral eukaryotic cell. Instead of being digested, this bacterium formed a mutually beneficial relationship with its host, eventually evolving into modern-day mitochondria.

This ancient association is evident in the structure of mitochondria:

1. **Double Membrane:** Mitochondria are enclosed in two membranes: an outer membrane that's porous and an inner membrane that's selectively permeable and extensively folded into structures called cristae. The intermembrane space between these layers holds a cocktail of enzymes.

2. **Mitochondrial DNA:** Unlike other cellular organelles, mitochondria have their own DNA (mtDNA) and can produce some of their proteins. This mtDNA is circular, reminiscent of bacterial genomes.

3. **Matrix:** The innermost compartment of the mitochondrion, the matrix, contains a variety of enzymes, mtDNA, and ribosomes. It's the site where several metabolic reactions, including some steps of cellular respiration, occur.

The Energetic Role: ATP Production

Mitochondria's reputation as cellular powerhouses is primarily due to their role in adenosine triphosphate (ATP) synthesis, the primary energy currency of the cell. Through a process called oxidative phosphorylation, mitochondria convert nutrients into ATP. This process involves a series of protein complexes in the inner mitochondrial membrane, collectively called the electron transport chain, which couples electron transfer to the pumping of protons, establishing a proton gradient. The enzyme ATP synthase utilizes this gradient to synthesize ATP from adenosine diphosphate (ADP) and inorganic phosphate.

Beyond Energy: Other Crucial Functions

1. **Calcium Homeostasis:** Mitochondria play a pivotal role in regulating intracellular calcium levels, which is crucial for various cellular processes including muscle contraction, neurotransmitter release, and cell signaling.

2. **Apoptosis:** Mitochondria are central players in programmed cell death, or apoptosis. In response to certain signals, they release cytochrome c, which activates a cascade of proteolytic enzymes leading to cell death.

3. **Biomolecule Synthesis:** Beyond energy production, the mitochondria are involved in synthesizing various biomolecules, including certain amino acids, iron-sulfur clusters, and heme groups.

Mitochondrial Dysfunction and Disease

Given their central role in energy production and other cellular processes, it's unsurprising that mitochondrial dysfunction is implicated in a plethora of diseases. From neurodegenerative disorders like Parkinson's and Alzheimer's to metabolic disorders such as diabetes, the health of the mitochondria is paramount. Additionally, mutations in mtDNA or genes involved in mitochondrial function can lead to a spectrum of mitochondrial diseases.

Conclusion

Mitochondria, with their bacterium-like origins, have evolved to become indispensable components of eukaryotic cells. Their roles stretch far beyond mere ATP production, influencing myriad cellular processes. As research continues to shed light on their complexities, it becomes ever clearer that maintaining mitochondrial health is fundamental to the overall health and vitality of an organism. As we move through the chapters of cellular biology, the significance of these powerhouses in aging and longevity will be further elucidated.

Mitochondrial Dysfunction and Its Links to Aging

Mitochondria, often dubbed the 'powerhouses' of the cell, are central to our understanding of aging and longevity. These dynamic organelles are not just mere energy producers; they influence a range of cellular functions from calcium homeostasis to programmed cell death. As cells age, the efficiency and functionality of mitochondria often decline, leading to what is broadly termed as 'mitochondrial dysfunction.' Unraveling the links between this dysfunction and aging offers promising insights into the biology of life's inevitable twilight.

The Cascade of Mitochondrial Dysfunction

Several events mark the descent of mitochondria into dysfunction:

1. **DNA Damage:** Mitochondrial DNA (mtDNA) is particularly susceptible to damage due to its close proximity to the electron transport chain, where reactive oxygen species (ROS) are generated. Unlike nuclear DNA, mtDNA lacks protective histones and has limited DNA repair mechanisms. Over time, accumulated mutations in mtDNA can impair the synthesis of essential proteins for oxidative phosphorylation.

2. **Reactive Oxygen Species (ROS):** While ROS are natural byproducts of the oxidative phosphorylation process, excessive ROS can damage cellular components, including proteins, lipids, and DNA.

Initially conceived as deleterious agents causing aging, ROS's role is now understood to be more nuanced, participating in signaling and adaptation. However, in elevated levels, they contribute to a vicious cycle where they cause mitochondrial damage and further ROS production.

3. **Decreased ATP Production:** As mitochondria become less efficient, their ability to produce ATP—the cell's energy currency—declines. This energy deficit can compromise various cellular processes, impacting cell health and function.

4. **Impaired Calcium Regulation:** Mitochondria help regulate intracellular calcium levels, essential for numerous cellular functions. Dysfunction can disrupt calcium homeostasis, contributing to cellular aging and susceptibility to external stressors.

Mitochondrial Dysfunction's Contribution to Aging

1. **Cell Senescence:** With declining mitochondrial efficiency and the accumulation of cellular damage, cells can enter a state of senescence. Senescent cells, although no longer dividing, remain metabolically active and often secrete pro-inflammatory factors that can negatively affect surrounding cells.

2. **Tissue Degeneration:** Tissues that heavily rely on energy, such as muscles and the brain, are particularly vulnerable to mitochondrial dysfunction. For instance, the progressive loss of mitochondrial function in neurons contributes to neurodegenerative diseases like Parkinson's and Alzheimer's.

3. **Stem Cell Exhaustion:** Stem cells, responsible for tissue regeneration, also rely on mitochondria for energy. A decline in mitochondrial function can exhaust the regenerative capacity of stem cells, impairing tissue repair and regeneration in aging organisms.

4. **Inflammation:** Dysfunctional mitochondria can trigger chronic inflammation through the release of damage-associated molecular patterns (DAMPs) and the aforementioned pro-inflammatory secretions from senescent cells.

Therapeutic Potential

The strong link between mitochondrial dysfunction and aging has spurred interest in therapeutic interventions. Approaches include:

- **Mitochondrial Antioxidants:** Compounds like MitoQ and SkQ1 are designed to target mitochondria and neutralize excessive ROS.
- **Mitochondrial Biogenesis Stimulators:** Compounds like resveratrol and SIRT1 activators can stimulate the formation of new mitochondria.
- **Mitophagy Enhancers:** Enhancing mitophagy, the process by which cells remove damaged mitochondria, can help maintain a healthy mitochondrial pool.

Conclusion

The intricate dance of life heavily depends on the rhythm set by mitochondria. As these organelles wane in function, the repercussions manifest in the aging process at cellular, tissue, and organismal levels. By understanding and potentially intervening in mitochondrial dysfunction, there's hope to ameliorate age-related decline, extending not just lifespan, but more crucially, healthspan—the period of life spent in good health.

The Role of Reactive Oxygen Species (ROS) in Cellular Function and Aging

Reactive Oxygen Species (ROS) often emerge in discussions surrounding cellular metabolism, aging, and disease. While the term may evoke images of unruly, damaging entities, ROS's role is far more nuanced, contributing to both physiological functions and pathological events. In the context of aging and mitochondrial function, understanding the dual nature of ROS provides a comprehensive view of their significance in cellular health and longevity.

What are ROS?

Reactive Oxygen Species are chemically reactive molecules containing oxygen. They arise mainly from the electron transport chain in mitochondria during aerobic respiration but can also originate from other enzymatic sources and external agents like radiation. Common ROS include superoxide anion (O_2^-), hydrogen peroxide (H_2O_2), and hydroxyl radicals ($\cdot OH$).

The Positive Side of ROS: Cellular Signaling and Defense

1. **Cellular Signaling:** ROS function as secondary messengers in various signaling pathways. They modulate the activity of several proteins and transcription factors, influencing processes from cell proliferation to differentiation. For instance, ROS-mediated activation of NF-κB can lead to the expression of genes involved in immunity and inflammation.

2. **Defense Against Pathogens:** In immune cells, like neutrophils, ROS production is dramatically upregulated to combat invading pathogens. This "respiratory burst" is a mechanism where ROS directly neutralize pathogens, playing a pivotal role in innate immunity.

3. **Adaptive Response:** At low or moderate levels, ROS can induce a cellular adaptive response, enhancing the cell's antioxidant defense system. This phenomenon, termed hormesis, is where mild stress promotes cellular adaptation, preparing the cell for more significant challenges.

The Dark Side of ROS: Damage and Dysregulation

1. **Oxidative Stress:** When the production of ROS overwhelms the cellular antioxidant defense systems, oxidative stress occurs. This imbalance leads to damage to DNA, proteins, and lipids, impairing their function and leading to potential mutations.

2. **Mitochondrial Damage:** ROS, especially when produced in excess within the mitochondria, can damage mitochondrial components, including mitochondrial DNA (mtDNA). Given that mtDNA encodes essential proteins for the electron transport chain, its damage can further elevate ROS production, creating a vicious cycle of dysfunction.

3. **Contribution to Disease:** Chronic oxidative stress, resulting from persistent elevated ROS levels, has been implicated in various diseases including neurodegenerative disorders (e.g., Parkinson's and Alzheimer's), cardiovascular diseases, cancers, and inflammatory conditions.

4. **Aging and Senescence:** There's a growing consensus that ROS, and the resulting oxidative stress, play a role in cellular aging. The accumulation of oxidative damage over time can trigger cellular senescence, a state of irreversible cell cycle arrest, which has implications for tissue function and regeneration.

ROS and Aging: The Mitochondrial Connection

The "Free Radical Theory of Aging" postulated by Denham Harman in the 1950s proposed that organisms age due to the accumulated damage inflicted by ROS. While this theory has evolved over the years, and aging is now understood to be multifactorial, ROS's role remains central. Mitochondrial dysfunction, leading to elevated ROS production, and the subsequent cellular damage, is considered a hallmark of aging.

Balancing ROS: Therapeutic Interventions

Given ROS's dual role, the goal isn't their elimination but achieving a balance:

1. **Antioxidants:** Compounds that neutralize ROS, such as vitamin C and E, are commonly known antioxidants. However, their effectiveness in vivo, especially concerning anti-aging, remains a topic of debate.

2. **Caloric Restriction:** Reduced calorie intake without malnutrition has been shown to reduce ROS production and extend lifespan in various organisms, pointing to a potential therapeutic avenue.

3. **Pharmacological Agents:** Drugs that target mitochondrial function and ROS production, such as metformin and NAD+ boosters, are under investigation for their potential anti-aging effects.

Conclusion

ROS, with their Jekyll and Hyde nature, exemplify the complexity of cellular processes. Far from being mere cellular byproducts, they play central roles in physiology and pathology alike. As our understanding of ROS deepens, it promises to illuminate paths to healthier aging and disease mitigation.

Chapter 5: DNA Damage and Repair

Mechanisms of DNA Damage: Unraveling the Assaults on the Blueprint of Life

The integrity of DNA, the molecule encoding the very essence of life, is under constant threat from various external and internal factors. Damage to this critical molecule is not only a fundamental cause for mutations leading to cancer but also plays a pivotal role in the aging process. Grasping the diverse mechanisms of DNA damage provides insight into the intricacies of cellular function, disease etiology, and longevity.

1. Oxidative Stress:

At the forefront of internal DNA damage is oxidative stress, primarily induced by reactive oxygen species (ROS). As byproducts of cellular metabolism, particularly during mitochondrial energy production, ROS can oxidize DNA bases, leading to modifications like 8-oxoguanine. If not correctly repaired, this can cause mispairing during DNA replication, leading to mutations.

2. UV Radiation:

Sunlight, though essential for life, carries the potential for DNA damage in the form of ultraviolet (UV) radiation. There are two primary types of DNA damage induced by UV light:

- *Cyclobutane Pyrimidine Dimers (CPDs):* When two adjacent pyrimidine bases (usually thymines) become covalently linked, impeding proper DNA replication and transcription.
- *6-4 Photoproducts:* A bond forms between the carbon-6 of one pyrimidine and the carbon-4 of an adjacent one.

Both these damages distort the DNA helix, and if left unrepaired, can result in mutations.

3. Ionizing Radiation:

Sources like X-rays and radioactive materials produce ionizing radiation that can cause single and double-strand breaks in the DNA. Double-strand breaks are particularly deleterious as they can lead to large scale chromosomal rearrangements if not accurately repaired.

4. Environmental Mutagens:

Various environmental chemicals, such as those in tobacco smoke (like benzo[a]pyrene) and industrial pollutants, can bind and modify DNA bases, leading to bulky DNA adducts. These adducts, if not excised, can block replication and transcription machinery, prompting mutations.

5. Spontaneous Hydrolysis:

Water, the very solvent of life, can occasionally betray DNA through spontaneous reactions. Hydrolysis can lead to the deamination of bases (e.g., cytosine to uracil) or the loss of purine bases, creating abasic sites. These sites become problematic during DNA replication.

6. DNA Replication Errors:

Even the sophisticated machinery of DNA replication isn't infallible. Errors during replication, though rare, can lead to mismatches, insertions, or deletions in the DNA sequence.

7. DNA Crosslinking:

Certain agents, both exogenous (like chemotherapeutic drugs) and endogenous (like malondialdehyde, a byproduct of lipid peroxidation), can induce covalent linkages between two DNA strands. This crosslinking obstructs DNA replication and transcription.

8. Topological Stress:

During DNA replication and transcription, the DNA can become overwound or underwound, leading to supercoiling. If not resolved, this topological stress can cause DNA breaks.

DNA Repair Mechanisms: The Cellular Safeguard

Understanding DNA damage is only half the story. Cells have evolved a suite of DNA repair mechanisms to address each type of damage:

- **Direct Repair:** Direct reversal of the damage without breaking the DNA backbone, such as in the case of O6-methylguanine.
- **Base Excision Repair (BER):** Removal and replacement of single damaged bases.
- **Nucleotide Excision Repair (NER):** Excision of a stretch of nucleotides containing the damage.
- **Mismatch Repair (MMR):** Corrects mismatches generated during DNA replication.
- **Double-strand Break Repair:** Through non-homologous end joining (NHEJ) or homologous recombination (HR).

Conclusion

The constancy of threats to DNA integrity underscores the delicate balance that life must maintain. As science delves deeper into the mechanisms of DNA damage and repair, potential avenues for intervention in disease progression and aging emerge, offering hope for extending healthspan and ensuring genomic integrity.

DNA Repair Pathways and Their Significance in Aging

The fabric of life, DNA, is under ceaseless threat from myriad sources, from the food we consume to the very air we breathe. Fortunately, cells are equipped with intricate repair systems that maintain the integrity of our genetic material. However, as with many biological processes, aging can influence the efficiency of these repair systems. Delving into the primary DNA repair pathways and their association with aging elucidates how preserving genetic fidelity affects longevity and healthspan.

1. Base Excision Repair (BER):

BER addresses small alterations to DNA bases, often resulting from oxidative stress or spontaneous hydrolysis. Enzymes like glycosylases detect and remove the aberrant base, after which other enzymes step in to fill the gap. A compromised BER pathway leads to the accumulation of mutations, which has been implicated in neurodegenerative diseases and aging-related cognitive decline.

2. Nucleotide Excision Repair (NER):

NER rectifies helix-distorting lesions, particularly those induced by ultraviolet radiation, such as thymine dimers. In NER, a stretch of DNA around the lesion is recognized and excised, and the gap filled using the complementary strand as a template. Deficiencies in NER are evident in conditions like xeroderma pigmentosum, where individuals are highly sensitive to UV radiation and display premature skin aging.

3. Mismatch Repair (MMR):

During DNA replication, occasional mismatches can occur. MMR systems recognize and correct these errors, ensuring high-fidelity replication. Impaired MMR elevates mutation rates and has been associated with certain cancers. Additionally, declining MMR efficiency with age may contribute to aging-associated genomic instability.

4. Double-strand Break Repair:

Arguably the most detrimental form of DNA damage, double-strand breaks (DSBs) are addressed through two primary pathways:

- **Non-homologous End Joining (NHEJ):** NHEJ directly ligates the broken ends of DNA, often resulting in small deletions or insertions. Due to its error-prone nature, excessive reliance on NHEJ can lead to genomic instability. Aging cells, with diminished capacity for the more precise homologous recombination, tend to resort to NHEJ, which may contribute to age-associated genetic anomalies.

- **Homologous Recombination (HR):** HR uses an intact sister chromatid as a template to repair the DSB, ensuring that the original sequence is restored. The efficiency of HR diminishes with age, leading to an increased reliance on the error-prone NHEJ.

5. Direct Repair:

Some lesions can be directly reversed without excising the base. For example, the enzyme O6-methylguanine-DNA methyltransferase directly repairs O6-methylguanine, a lesion formed due to exposure to certain alkylating agents.

Significance in Aging

As organisms age, several interconnected phenomena occur:

- **Accumulation of DNA Damage:** Due to prolonged exposure to environmental mutagens and the inherent errors in cellular processes, older cells tend to have more DNA damage.

- **Decline in Repair Efficiency:** The machinery responsible for DNA repair exhibits reduced efficiency with age, leading to a higher likelihood of retaining DNA damage.

- **Cellular Senescence and Apoptosis:** Accumulated DNA damage can push cells into a state of permanent growth arrest (senescence) or programmed cell death (apoptosis). Both processes are protective against cancer but can contribute to tissue dysfunction, a hallmark of aging.

- **Cancer Susceptibility:** Reduced DNA repair capacity increases the risk of mutations, elevating cancer susceptibility in older individuals.

Conclusion

Understanding the interplay between DNA repair and aging provides valuable insights into the processes that underpin health and longevity. The gradual decline in the efficiency of DNA repair mechanisms may not only serve as a biomarker of aging but also present a potential target for interventions to enhance healthspan. Preserving the integrity of our DNA, the very foundation of life, is paramount to aging gracefully and staving off age-associated diseases.

The Relationship between DNA Damage, Mutations, and Age-Related Diseases

DNA, often termed the blueprint of life, holds the intricate instructions that guide the synthesis and function of proteins, as well as the regulation and maintenance of cellular activities. Over time, this blueprint, like any heavily used manuscript, may become worn, bearing the marks of accumulated damage. DNA damage, if not effectively repaired, can lead to mutations, alterations in the sequence of DNA. This relationship between DNA damage, mutations, and the onset of age-related diseases is a profound exploration into the interconnectedness of cellular events and the phenotypic manifestations of aging.

1. DNA Damage: The Initial Blow

Various agents and circumstances inflict damage on DNA. These include external factors like UV radiation, chemical mutagens, and ionizing radiation. Simultaneously, internal factors, such as metabolic byproducts (e.g., reactive oxygen species) and replication errors, can also harm DNA. Over time, with the continuous onslaught from these agents, DNA damage accumulates, particularly if the cellular repair mechanisms become less efficient or overwhelmed.

2. From Damage to Mutation

While cells possess intricate systems to detect and rectify DNA damage, no system is infallible. Repair mechanisms can sometimes make errors, or particular damage can escape the cellular surveillance system altogether. When damaged DNA is replicated, it can lead to mutations: changes in the nucleotide sequence. These mutations, if located in crucial regions of the genome, such as protein-coding sequences or regulatory regions, can have detrimental functional implications.

3. Age-Related Diseases: A Web of Mutations

The manifestation of mutations in vital genes can lead to the onset of age-related diseases:

- **Cancer:** Perhaps the most direct link between DNA damage, mutations, and disease is seen in cancer. Mutations in genes that regulate cell growth, division, or DNA repair can lead to uncontrolled cell proliferation. As individuals age, the likelihood of accumulating such mutations increases, explaining the higher incidence of cancer in older populations.

- **Neurodegenerative Diseases:** Conditions like Alzheimer's and Parkinson's disease have been associated with DNA damage, particularly in the mitochondrial DNA. Mutations in the mitochondrial genome can compromise cellular energy production, a critical factor for neurons given their high energy demand.

- **Cardiovascular Diseases:** Atherosclerosis, leading to conditions like heart attacks and strokes, has been linked to DNA damage. Endothelial dysfunction, inflammation, and oxidative stress can lead to DNA damage, mutations, and cellular senescence, all contributing to the progression of vascular diseases.

- **Immunosenescence:** The immune system's efficiency wanes with age, a phenomenon termed immunosenescence. DNA damage and mutations in immune cells can impair their function, rendering older individuals more susceptible to infections and reducing vaccine efficacy.

4. Feedback Loops: Disease Enhancing DNA Damage

Age-related diseases themselves can exacerbate DNA damage, creating a vicious cycle. For instance, the inflammatory environment in atherosclerotic plaques can enhance oxidative stress, leading to further DNA damage. Similarly, neurodegenerative conditions can compromise cellular maintenance systems, amplifying DNA damage in neuronal cells.

Conclusion

The relationship between DNA damage, mutations, and age-related diseases paints a vivid picture of the cellular events that underlie the physiological and pathological aspects of aging. As the intricate dance of cellular processes plays out over the years, DNA bears the brunt of the wear and tear, leading to the emergence of diseases that mark the aging phenotype.

Deciphering this relationship provides not only insights into the biology of aging but also potential therapeutic avenues. Interventions targeting DNA repair or mitigating DNA damage could potentially delay, if not prevent, the onset of age-related diseases, paving the way for a healthier, more extended period of life.

Chapter 6: Cellular Senescence

What is Cellular Senescence?

Cellular senescence, a term derived from the Latin word "senex" meaning "old man" or "old age," is a biological phenomenon wherein a cell permanently loses its ability to divide and proliferate, entering a state of irreversible growth arrest. While cellular senescence plays crucial roles in embryonic development and tissue repair, it is also intrinsically linked to the aging process and age-associated pathologies. Understanding the essence of cellular senescence offers a glimpse into the mechanisms that underpin organismal aging and the strategies to counteract its detrimental effects.

1. Discovery and Initial Observations:

The concept of cellular senescence was first introduced in the early 1960s when Leonard Hayflick observed that human fibroblasts, grown in culture, had a limited replicative lifespan. After a certain number of divisions, these cells entered a state of irreversible growth arrest, a phenomenon later termed the 'Hayflick Limit.' This discovery debunked the prevailing notion that cells were immortal in culture, setting the stage for further exploration into the molecular underpinnings of this process.

2. Triggers of Cellular Senescence:

A plethora of stimuli can drive a cell into senescence:

- **Replicative Senescence:** As cells divide, telomeres, the protective caps at the ends of chromosomes, shorten. Once telomeres reach a critically short length, they can trigger replicative senescence.
- **Oncogene-Induced Senescence:** Activation of certain oncogenes can thrust cells into a senescent state, a mechanism that serves as a protective barrier against malignant transformation.
- **DNA Damage:** Persistent DNA damage, whether due to external mutagens or errors in DNA replication, can initiate cellular senescence. This response serves as a protective measure, preventing

the proliferation of damaged cells that might otherwise give rise to tumors.

- **Other Stressors:** Factors such as oxidative stress, mitochondrial dysfunction, and even certain therapeutic agents can induce cellular senescence.

3. Characteristics of Senescent Cells:

While senescent cells cease to divide, they remain metabolically active and undergo various morphological and biochemical changes:

- **Enlarged Morphology:** Senescent cells often become flattened and enlarged.

- **Senescence-Associated β-galactosidase (SA-β-gal):** This enzyme, active at pH 6.0, is a hallmark of senescent cells and serves as a widely-used marker for detecting them.

- **Senescence-Associated Secretory Phenotype (SASP):** Senescent cells secrete a plethora of cytokines, growth factors, and proteases, collectively termed SASP. While SASP factors can have beneficial effects, such as in wound healing, they can also promote inflammation, tissue dysfunction, and even cancer progression.

4. Role in Aging and Disease:

Senescent cells accumulate in tissues with age. While they serve beneficial roles, their persistence can be deleterious:

- **Tissue Dysfunction:** The SASP can disrupt tissue architecture and function, contributing to age-associated tissue decline.

- **Inflammation:** Senescent cells can instigate chronic inflammation, a key driver of various age-related diseases, including cardiovascular diseases and neurodegenerative disorders.

- **Cancer:** Paradoxically, while cellular senescence is a protective mechanism against cancer, the SASP can create an environment conducive to cancer progression.

5. Therapeutic Implications:

The discovery of the detrimental effects of accumulated senescent cells has led to the idea of "senolytics" – drugs that selectively eliminate senescent cells. By purging tissues of these cells, it is hypothesized that one can ameliorate age-associated pathologies and potentially extend healthspan.

Conclusion

Cellular senescence, a double-edged sword, is both a guardian and a nemesis. While it shields against early-life tumorigenesis and aids in tissue repair, its persistent effects contribute to the tapestry of aging. Understanding and harnessing this knowledge opens doors to innovative strategies for promoting healthy aging and combatting age-associated diseases.

Triggers and Markers of Senescence

Cellular senescence, once merely a cellular curiosity observed in culture dishes, has now been recognized as a fundamental biological process with deep implications for aging, tissue repair, and disease. The pivotal questions that researchers grapple with are: What drives a cell into this state? And, once there, how can we accurately identify senescent cells in the body? The answers to these questions lie in understanding the triggers and markers of senescence.

1. Triggers of Cellular Senescence:

Several factors can push a cell into the senescent state, acting as molecular tripwires:

- **Telomere Attrition:** Telomeres, the protective end caps of chromosomes, shorten with every cell division. When they reach a critically short length, they can no longer safeguard the chromosome ends, triggering a DNA damage response that leads to senescence. This phenomenon is termed replicative senescence.
- **Oncogene Activation:** The activation of oncogenes, which are genes that have the potential to transform a cell into a tumor cell,

can induce senescence. This mechanism, called oncogene-induced senescence (OIS), serves as a fail-safe, preventing cells with oncogenic mutations from proliferating uncontrollably.

- **DNA Damage:** Exogenous factors like radiation or chemicals, as well as endogenous processes like oxidative stress, can damage DNA. Persistent, unresolved DNA damage can push cells into a senescent state, serving as a protective mechanism to halt the propagation of damaged DNA.

- **Mitochondrial Dysfunction:** Mitochondria, the cellular powerhouses, have been implicated in senescence. Dysfunctional mitochondria can induce oxidative stress and metabolic changes that activate senescence pathways.

2. Markers of Cellular Senescence:

To delineate and study senescent cells in tissues, researchers have identified several hallmark features:

- **Senescence-Associated β-galactosidase (SA-β-gal):** A characteristic enzyme activity seen in senescent cells, SA-β-gal functions at pH 6.0 and remains one of the most widely used markers. However, its presence alone is not definitive proof of senescence, as other non-senescent cells can also exhibit this activity under certain conditions.

- **Cell Cycle Inhibitors:** Proteins such as p16^INK4a and p21^CIP1/WAF1, which inhibit the cell cycle machinery, are often upregulated in senescent cells. These inhibitors block the progression of the cell cycle, cementing the cell in its non-dividing state.

- **Senescence-Associated Secretory Phenotype (SASP):** One of the most defining features of senescent cells is the SASP – a cocktail of cytokines, chemokines, growth factors, and proteases that senescent cells release. While the exact composition can vary based on the senescence trigger and cell type, certain factors like interleukin-6 (IL-6) and interleukin-8 (IL-8) are frequently upregulated.

- **DNA Damage Response (DDR) Foci:** Since many senescence triggers revolve around DNA damage, the presence of DDR foci, visible aggregations of DNA damage response proteins at sites of DNA lesions, is a common feature of senescent cells.

- **Telomere Dysfunction:** Telomere-associated foci (TAF) and dysfunctional telomere-induced foci (TIF) can be observed in senescent cells experiencing telomere dysfunction.

Conclusion

Understanding the triggers and markers of cellular senescence provides tools and insights to decipher the mosaic of aging and age-related diseases. By recognizing what propels cells into senescence and being able to identify them once they're there, researchers can begin to address the broader questions: How do senescent cells contribute to aging? And can we therapeutically target these cells to ameliorate age-associated decline? These queries underline the profound significance of understanding the triggers and markers of this intriguing cellular state.

The Role of Senescent Cells in Tissue Aging and Regeneration

Cellular senescence, with its inherent growth arrest and distinctive secretory profile, plays multifaceted roles in the orchestration of tissue aging and regeneration. As with many biological phenomena, the effects of senescent cells are double-edged: they have the potential to both harm and heal. By delving into the roles these cells play, we can gain a more comprehensive understanding of the complexities of aging and tissue repair.

1. Senescent Cells in Tissue Aging:

Senescent cells accumulate in tissues over time, and their presence is a hallmark of aging tissues. Here's how they contribute to the aging process:

- **Senescence-Associated Secretory Phenotype (SASP):** Senescent cells release a plethora of molecules, including cytokines, growth factors, and proteases, known as the SASP. While some SASP factors can be beneficial, many have pro-inflammatory properties, leading to chronic inflammation in tissues—a key driver of many age-related diseases.

- **Tissue Dysfunction:** The SASP can disrupt the normal architecture and function of tissues. For instance, in the skin, an accumulation of senescent cells can lead to decreased dermal thickness, reduced collagen content, and impaired wound healing.

- **Stem Cell Dysfunction:** Senescent cells can negatively influence stem cell niches, impairing the function and proliferative capacity of stem cells. This can lead to diminished tissue repair and regeneration capabilities as we age.

2. Senescent Cells in Tissue Regeneration:

Paradoxically, while senescent cells are often detrimental in the context of aging, they can play a positive role in tissue repair and regeneration:

- **Short-Term Benefits of the SASP:** In the immediate aftermath of tissue injury, the SASP can be beneficial. The released factors can recruit immune cells to the injury site, clear damaged cells, and stimulate tissue repair. For example, after a skin wound, the SASP can promote fibroblast proliferation and collagen deposition, aiding in wound closure.

- **Stem Cell Modulation:** In certain contexts, senescent cells can release factors that stimulate stem cells to divide and differentiate, enhancing tissue regeneration. This has been observed in the liver, where senescent cells can promote liver regeneration following partial hepatectomy.

- **Tumor Suppression:** One of the primary reasons cells enter senescence is to prevent the proliferation of damaged or mutated cells that might give rise to tumors. In this sense, senescence acts as a natural tumor suppressor mechanism, halting the growth of potential cancer cells and often leading to their clearance by the immune system.

3. Balancing the Scales:

Given the dual roles of senescent cells, the challenge lies in determining how to harness their beneficial effects while mitigating their detrimental ones:

- **Timely Clearance:** One strategy is to facilitate the timely clearance of senescent cells after they've performed their beneficial roles. If senescent cells are removed before they accumulate to detrimental levels, it could prevent their adverse effects on tissues.
- **Modulating the SASP:** If researchers can modify the SASP to retain its beneficial factors while eliminating the harmful ones, senescent cells could be transformed into purely regenerative agents without the aging side effects.

Conclusion

The intricate dance of senescent cells in the arenas of tissue aging and regeneration underscores the beauty and complexity of biology. These cells, once seen as mere bystanders of the aging process, are now at the forefront of research in rejuvenation and regenerative medicine. By understanding their roles and learning to modulate their effects, we inch closer to unlocking strategies to promote healthy aging and efficient tissue repair.

Chapter 7: Autophagy and Protein Homeostasis

The Importance of Protein Quality Control

At its core, life is orchestrated by an intricate interplay of proteins, which function as the workhorses of the cell, executing a myriad of tasks that sustain cellular health and functionality. However, these proteins are not infallible. They can become damaged, misfolded, or may sometimes be produced erroneously. The consequences of unchecked faulty proteins can be dire, leading to cellular dysfunction, diseases, and aging. Enter the role of protein quality control – the cellular safeguard ensuring proteins are correctly folded and functional.

1. Protein Folding and Its Challenges:

The functionality of a protein is intrinsically tied to its three-dimensional shape. Following their synthesis on ribosomes, proteins fold into specific configurations, guided by their amino acid sequences. Yet, this process can be error-prone. Influences such as genetic mutations, environmental stressors, or cellular aging can lead to misfolded proteins.

Misfolded proteins are problematic for several reasons:

- They can lose their intended function, leading to a deficit in crucial cellular activities.
- They can aggregate, forming toxic clumps that disrupt cellular homeostasis.
- Their presence can indicate or lead to broader cellular stress, as seen in neurodegenerative diseases like Alzheimer's or Parkinson's, where protein aggregates are hallmark features.

2. The Protein Quality Control System:

To combat the challenges of protein misfolding, cells have evolved a robust protein quality control system. This system comprises a network of molecular chaperones and proteolytic machines.

- **Molecular Chaperones:** These are proteins that assist in the folding or refolding of other proteins. They don't get incorporated into the final structure but act as guides, ensuring the correct folding process. Examples include the heat shock proteins (Hsps), which are upregulated in response to cellular stress and help refold or stabilize damaged proteins.

- **Proteolytic Machines:** If a protein is irreparably damaged or misfolded, it's tagged for destruction. The two primary proteolytic systems in the cell are the proteasome and the lysosome. The ubiquitin-proteasome pathway tags damaged proteins with ubiquitin chains, signaling them for degradation by the proteasome. Lysosomes, on the other hand, degrade proteins through autophagy, a process wherein cellular components are encapsulated and delivered to the lysosome for destruction.

3. Protein Quality Control in Aging and Disease:

The efficiency of the protein quality control system isn't static; it diminishes with age. This decline is believed to contribute to the aging process and the onset of age-related diseases.

- As the quality control mechanisms wane, there's an accumulation of misfolded or aggregated proteins, which can interfere with cellular functions and lead to cellular senescence or cell death.

- Many neurodegenerative diseases are characterized by the presence of protein aggregates, indicating a failure in the protein quality control pathways. For example, Alzheimer's is associated with amyloid-beta plaques, and Parkinson's with alpha-synuclein aggregates.

4. Therapeutic Potential:

Understanding the protein quality control system offers avenues for therapeutic interventions. By boosting the activity of chaperones or enhancing proteolytic degradation, it might be possible to mitigate the effects of protein misfolding diseases or even delay aspects of the aging process.

Conclusion

The protein quality control system is a testament to the cell's commitment to precision and efficiency. As we continue to understand its intricacies and nuances, we not only unravel the mysteries of cellular health but also uncover potential strategies to combat some of the most challenging diseases of our time. In essence, the fidelity of the proteome, overseen by this system, is foundational to life's continuity and vitality.

Mechanisms of Autophagy and Its Role in Longevity

Autophagy, a term derived from the Greek words for "self" and "eating," is a cellular process that facilitates the degradation and recycling of cellular components. Over the past few decades, the role of autophagy in health, disease, and notably, longevity, has become an area of intense scientific exploration. As our understanding of this process deepens, its significance in the biology of aging becomes increasingly evident.

1. Mechanisms of Autophagy:

At its core, autophagy is the cell's housekeeping mechanism. It cleans up cellular debris, damaged organelles, and misfolded proteins by enveloping them in a double-membraned structure called an autophagosome. The autophagosome then fuses with a lysosome, a cellular organelle filled with digestive enzymes, resulting in the breakdown of the enclosed materials. The resulting breakdown products, such as amino acids and fatty acids, are then recycled back into the cell's metabolism.

Autophagy is regulated by a series of complex signaling pathways, with the mTOR (mechanistic target of rapamycin) pathway playing a pivotal role. Under nutrient-rich conditions, mTOR is active and suppresses autophagy. However, in conditions of cellular stress or nutrient deprivation, mTOR activity is reduced, leading to the activation of autophagy.

2. Autophagy in Longevity:

The link between autophagy and longevity is supported by numerous studies across different organisms. Here's how autophagy contributes to a longer, healthier life:

- **Cellular Maintenance:** Regular cleanup of damaged organelles and proteins ensures that cellular processes run smoothly. For instance, by removing damaged mitochondria, autophagy prevents the accumulation of reactive oxygen species, which are associated with cellular aging.
- **Protection Against Neurodegenerative Diseases:** Many neurodegenerative diseases, such as Alzheimer's and Parkinson's, are characterized by the accumulation of protein aggregates. Autophagy aids in clearing these aggregates, thus offering a protective effect against such diseases.
- **Promotion of Stem Cell Function:** Autophagy is crucial for the maintenance and differentiation of stem cells, which are essential for tissue regeneration. As we age, the ability of tissues to regenerate diminishes, but efficient autophagy can help maintain robust stem cell functions.
- **Metabolic Benefits:** Autophagy helps in lipid metabolism, reducing the accumulation of fat droplets in cells. It also plays a role in glycemic control, thereby offering protection against metabolic disorders.

3. Caloric Restriction, Autophagy, and Longevity:

One of the most consistent interventions known to extend lifespan across multiple organisms is caloric restriction (CR)–a reduction in calorie intake without malnutrition. One of the mechanisms through which CR confers its longevity benefits is believed to be the activation of autophagy. As nutrient intake is reduced, the mTOR pathway is inhibited, leading to the upregulation of autophagy. This increased autophagic activity facilitates cellular maintenance and promotes healthspan.

4. Future Perspectives and Therapeutic Potential:

Given the clear benefits of autophagy in promoting health and longevity, there's keen interest in developing interventions that can modulate autophagy. Drugs like rapamycin, which inhibit the mTOR pathway, have been shown to extend lifespan in various organisms. Moreover, other natural compounds, like resveratrol and spermidine, have also been identified as potential autophagy enhancers.

Conclusion

Autophagy stands at the nexus of cellular health, aging, and longevity. By understanding its mechanisms and roles, scientists hope to harness its potential to promote longer, healthier lives. As we move forward, the intricate dance of autophagy continues to reveal fascinating insights into the biology of life and the passage of time.

The Impact of Proteostasis Disruption in Aging

Proteostasis, a portmanteau of "protein" and "homeostasis," represents the complex network of processes that cells utilize to maintain a balanced and functional protein environment. This includes protein synthesis, folding, trafficking, and degradation. Maintaining proteostasis is essential for cellular health and function, and disruptions in this equilibrium have been intrinsically linked to aging and age-related diseases. As we age, the machinery that governs proteostasis becomes less efficient, leading to a cascade of consequences that can adversely impact health and lifespan.

1. The Proteostasis Network:

The proteostasis network comprises three primary components:

- **Chaperones and co-chaperones:** These molecules assist in the folding and refolding of proteins, ensuring they achieve and maintain their functional three-dimensional configurations.
- **Ubiquitin-proteasome system (UPS):** This is the primary pathway for the degradation of misfolded, damaged, or redundant proteins. Proteins marked for destruction are tagged with ubiquitin molecules and subsequently degraded by the proteasome.

- **Autophagy-lysosomal pathway:** This pathway involves the sequestration of cellular components, including proteins, in membrane-bound vesicles that fuse with lysosomes for degradation.

2. Disruption of Proteostasis in Aging:

Aging is accompanied by a decline in the efficiency of the proteostasis network. Several factors contribute to this decline:

- **Reduced chaperone function:** As cells age, the function and expression of molecular chaperones decrease, leading to an accumulation of misfolded proteins.
- **Compromised proteasomal activity:** The efficiency of the UPS diminishes with age, hindering the cell's ability to degrade unwanted proteins.
- **Impaired autophagy:** The autophagy-lysosomal pathway becomes less active in older cells, leading to an accumulation of damaged organelles and protein aggregates.

3. Consequences of Proteostasis Disruption:

The repercussions of a disturbed proteostasis network in aging are vast:

- **Protein aggregation:** Accumulation of misfolded or damaged proteins can lead to their aggregation. These aggregates can be toxic, disrupting cellular processes and functions. For example, the aggregates found in Alzheimer's disease (amyloid-beta plaques) or Parkinson's disease (Lewy bodies) are symptomatic of proteostasis failure.
- **Cellular stress:** Disruptions in proteostasis can induce endoplasmic reticulum (ER) stress, activating the unfolded protein response (UPR). Chronic activation of the UPR can lead to inflammation, another hallmark of aging.
- **Decreased cellular functionality:** As the proteostasis machinery becomes compromised, cells are less able to perform their designated functions, leading to tissue and organ dysfunction.

4. Proteostasis, Longevity, and Age-related Diseases:

Disruption in proteostasis is not merely a consequence of aging but can also be a driver of the aging process itself. Interventions that enhance proteostasis mechanisms, such as caloric restriction or the modulation of specific signaling pathways, have been shown to extend lifespan in various organisms.

Furthermore, the collapse of proteostasis is a shared feature among numerous age-related diseases, particularly neurodegenerative disorders. Restoring or bolstering proteostasis has become a therapeutic target for combating these diseases.

Conclusion

Proteostasis represents one of the critical pillars of cellular function and health. As the guardians of the proteome, the intricate networks that oversee protein homeostasis play a decisive role in the trajectory of aging. Understanding the nexus between proteostasis and aging offers a promising avenue for interventions that might ameliorate age-associated declines and extend healthy human lifespans. The quest to unravel the complexities of proteostasis and harness its potential continues to be one of the most exciting frontiers in the biology of aging.

Chapter 8: The Role of Epigenetics in Aging

Introduction to Epigenetics and Its Mechanisms

In the vast realm of genetics, the actual DNA sequence — the series of nucleotides that spell out our genetic code — represents just the tip of the iceberg. Beyond this "text" lies a complex layer of regulation, determining which genes are turned on or off, under what circumstances, and to what extent. This regulatory layer, which influences gene expression without altering the underlying DNA sequence, is the focus of epigenetics.

1. What is Epigenetics?

The term "epigenetics" is derived from the Greek prefix "epi-", meaning "above" or "over", suggesting a layer atop genetics. Epigenetics refers to changes in gene activity that do not involve alterations to the underlying DNA sequence. These changes can be inherited, and they can also be influenced by environmental factors, experiences, and even individual choices, such as diet or exposure to toxins.

2. Key Epigenetic Mechanisms:

The primary mechanisms of epigenetic regulation include DNA methylation, histone modification, and RNA-associated silencing. Each of these processes influences how genes are expressed in cells.

- **DNA Methylation:** This is perhaps the most studied epigenetic mechanism. It involves the addition of a methyl group to the DNA molecule, usually at a cytosine nucleotide. When methyl groups are added to a particular gene, that gene is turned off or "silenced". DNA methylation is crucial for processes such as embryonic development, genomic imprinting, and X-chromosome inactivation.
- **Histone Modification:** DNA in cells is not loose; it's wound around proteins called histones. Together, DNA and histones

form a structure called chromatin. The way DNA is wound around these histones can change, making genes more or less accessible for transcription. Histones can be modified through the addition or removal of specific chemical groups, including methyl, acetyl, and phosphate groups. Depending on the type of modification and its location, gene expression can be upregulated or down-regulated.

- **RNA-associated Silencing:** Another mechanism of epigenetic regulation involves small non-coding RNA molecules. These molecules can target specific sequences of DNA and influence their activity, typically resulting in gene silencing. The RNA-induced silencing complex (RISC) is a key player in this process.

3. Why Epigenetics is Important:

Epigenetic changes play a pivotal role in development and differentiation. For instance, while a neuron and a liver cell have the same DNA, their different functions and characteristics are the result of distinct patterns of gene expression, influenced significantly by epigenetic factors.

Moreover, epigenetic changes are reversible, making them potential targets for therapeutic interventions. Epigenetic dysregulation has been implicated in a myriad of diseases, including various cancers, mental disorders, and age-related conditions.

4. Epigenetics, Environment, and Lifestyle:

An intriguing aspect of epigenetics is its responsiveness to external factors. Environmental triggers, including diet, stress, exposure to toxins, and even behaviors like smoking, can induce epigenetic changes. For instance, studies on identical twins have shown that while they start with almost identical epigenomes, these can diverge significantly over their lifetimes, based on their individual experiences and choices.

Conclusion

Epigenetics introduces a dynamic perspective to the traditionally static view of genetics. The understanding that there's a flexible layer of genetic regulation, sensitive to our environment and lifestyle, underscores the profound interplay between nature and nurture. As we continue to decode the intricacies of epigenetic mechanisms, we stand on the threshold of significant breakthroughs, not only in comprehending the essence of life and development but also in devising innovative therapeutic approaches to combat diseases and age-related challenges.

How Epigenetic Changes Influence the Aging Process

Aging is a multifaceted phenomenon, driven by a myriad of interconnected factors. While the role of genetics in aging has been extensively studied, the intricate dance of epigenetics adds another layer of complexity to the narrative. Over time, our epigenome – the collection of chemical compounds that tell our genome what to do – undergoes significant changes. These epigenetic modifications influence the aging process, shaping how we age and our susceptibility to age-related diseases.

1. The Epigenetic Clock and Aging:

One of the most groundbreaking discoveries in epigenetic research is the concept of the 'epigenetic clock.' Researchers identified specific patterns of DNA methylation that correlate with chronological age. Incredibly, by assessing these methylation patterns, scientists can predict an individual's age with remarkable accuracy. More intriguingly, deviations between the predicted 'epigenetic age' and the actual chronological age can provide insights into an individual's health and longevity. For instance, an accelerated epigenetic age compared to the chronological age might indicate an increased risk of age-related diseases and mortality.

2. Epigenetic Drift and Aging:

As we age, the epigenetic landscape of our cells tends to shift, a phenomenon termed 'epigenetic drift.' This results in a gradual loss of the tightly regulated epigenetic patterns observed in youth. Such drift can lead to genes being inappropriately turned on or off, which can disrupt cellular function and increase the risk of diseases. Interestingly, identical twins, who share the same genetic makeup, show increasing epigenetic divergence as they age, emphasizing the role of environmental and stochastic factors in shaping the epigenome.

3. Epigenetic Changes and Age-related Diseases:

There's a close link between epigenetic alterations and various age-related diseases:

- **Cancer:** Epigenetic changes can activate oncogenes or silence tumor suppressor genes, promoting cancer development and progression.
- **Neurodegenerative Diseases:** Conditions like Alzheimer's and Parkinson's disease have been associated with specific epigenetic modifications, impacting genes vital for neuronal function and health.
- **Cardiovascular Diseases:** Epigenetic changes can influence genes related to inflammation, cholesterol metabolism, and blood pressure regulation, all crucial players in cardiovascular health.

4. Lifestyle, Environment, and Epigenetic Aging:

External factors play a pivotal role in dictating epigenetic changes associated with aging:

- **Diet:** Nutritional choices can influence DNA methylation patterns and histone modifications, potentially accelerating or decelerating aging.
- **Stress:** Chronic stress has been shown to induce specific epigenetic alterations, impacting genes associated with stress response, inflammation, and cellular health.
- **Environmental Toxins:** Exposure to certain toxins and pollutants can lead to persistent epigenetic changes, which may contribute to accelerated aging and heightened disease risk.

5. The Promise of Epigenetic Interventions:

Given the reversible nature of epigenetic marks, there's considerable interest in developing interventions that target the epigenome to counteract age-related changes and diseases. Drugs that modulate DNA methylation or histone modifications are already being used or trialled for specific diseases, particularly cancers. There's hope that similar strategies might be employed to delay aging or mitigate its associated challenges.

Conclusion

The exploration of the epigenetic landscape offers a fresh perspective on the age-old quest to understand aging. By uncovering how our lifestyles and environments leave lasting marks on our genome's functionality without changing its code, we gain deeper insights into the aging process and the factors that shape it. As we advance in our epigenetic journey, the dream of harnessing this knowledge to enhance healthspan and perhaps even lifespan seems ever more plausible.

Potential Therapeutic Interventions Targeting the Epigenome

As our understanding of the intricacies of epigenetics has grown, so too has the realization of its vast therapeutic potential. The ability of epigenetic modifications to regulate gene expression without changing the DNA sequence itself presents a unique opportunity. Unlike mutations in the DNA sequence, which are challenging to reverse, epigenetic changes are potentially reversible. Consequently, the epigenome is emerging as a promising target for interventions in a range of diseases, including cancer, neurodegenerative disorders, and metabolic diseases. Here, we explore the budding realm of epigenetic therapeutic interventions.

1. DNA Methylation Modulators:

Hypermethylation of gene promoter regions, leading to the silencing of tumor suppressor genes, is a frequent event in many cancers. Drugs that inhibit DNA methyltransferases, the enzymes responsible for adding methyl groups to DNA, can reverse this hypermethylation.

- **Azacitidine** and **Decitabine** are two FDA-approved drugs for the treatment of myelodysplastic syndromes (a group of bone marrow disorders). They work by incorporating themselves into the DNA and trapping DNA methyltransferases, leading to the enzymes' degradation and subsequent hypomethylation.

2. Histone Modification Modulators:

Histone modifications play a central role in gene regulation. Abnormal histone modifications can lead to inappropriate gene silencing or activation.

- **Histone Deacetylase Inhibitors (HDACi):** These are a class of drugs that inhibit histone deacetylases, enzymes that remove acetyl groups from histones. By inhibiting these enzymes, HDACi promote a more open chromatin structure and reactivate silenced genes. Vorinostat and Romidepsin are two HDACi approved for the treatment of cutaneous T-cell lymphoma.
- **Bromodomain Inhibitors:** Bromodomains recognize and bind to acetylated histones, influencing gene expression. Inhibitors targeting bromodomains, especially the BET family, are under investigation for their potential in treating various cancers.

3. RNA-Based Therapies:

Small non-coding RNAs, especially microRNAs (miRNAs), are influential epigenetic regulators. Dysregulated miRNA expression can lead to diseases.

- **MiRNA Mimics and AntagomiRs:** These are synthetic RNA molecules designed to mimic endogenous miRNAs or inhibit their activity, respectively. They're being explored as therapeutic agents for cancers, cardiovascular diseases, and hepatic disorders.

4. Epigenetic Diet and Nutraceuticals:

Dietary components can modulate epigenetic marks. For instance:

- **Genistein**, found in soy, can influence DNA methylation patterns.
- **Sulforaphane**, present in cruciferous vegetables, has been shown to inhibit HDACs.

- **Curcumin**, from turmeric, affects both DNA methylation and histone modifications.

The idea of an 'epigenetic diet', rich in such compounds, is being explored for its potential in disease prevention and health promotion.

5. Epigenetic Editing:

Using CRISPR/Cas9 technology, it's now possible to target specific genomic locations and introduce or remove epigenetic marks. This 'epigenome editing' holds enormous potential for precision medicine, allowing tailored interventions at the gene level.

6. Challenges and the Way Forward:

While the potential of epigenetic therapies is immense, challenges remain. Epigenetic drugs often have a broad spectrum of activity, which can lead to off-target effects. The development of more selective, targeted agents is an active research area. Additionally, the plasticity of the epigenome, while a therapeutic opportunity, can also be a hurdle, as epigenetic states can revert, necessitating sustained interventions.

Conclusion

The epigenome, with its dynamic and reversible nature, offers a novel and promising frontier in therapeutics. As we delve deeper into the complexities of epigenetic regulation and its perturbations in diseases, the prospect of 'epigenetic therapies'—once a distant dream—is becoming an impending reality. With continued research and innovation, we stand on the cusp of harnessing the epigenome's potential to revolutionize medicine and health care.

Chapter 9: Inflammation and Aging

Chronic Inflammation as a Hallmark of Aging

Aging is a complex, multifaceted process characterized by the gradual decline in physiological functions, leading to increased susceptibility to diseases and eventually death. While many factors contribute to aging, one of the most recognized and studied hallmarks is chronic inflammation. Often termed "inflammaging," this low-grade, persistent inflammatory state is intricately linked with the aging process and various age-related pathologies.

1. What is Inflammaging?

The term "inflammaging" was coined to describe the chronic, low-grade inflammation observed in older individuals in the absence of overt infection. Unlike acute inflammation, which is a rapid, protective response to injury or pathogens, inflammaging is a smoldering process, typically not severe enough to cause immediate symptoms but sufficiently intense to contribute to age-related tissue damage over time.

2. Causes of Inflammaging:

Several factors contribute to the onset and persistence of inflammaging:

- **Cellular Senescence:** As cells age, they can enter a state of senescence, where they no longer divide but remain metabolically active. These senescent cells release a plethora of inflammatory mediators, known as the senescence-associated secretory phenotype (SASP), which can perpetuate the inflammatory environment.

- **Mitochondrial Dysfunction:** With age, mitochondria, the cellular powerhouses, can become less efficient and leaky. This can result in the release of reactive oxygen species (ROS) and mitochondrial DNA, both of which can trigger inflammatory responses.

- **Dysregulated Immune System:** Aging is associated with a decline in immune function, termed immunosenescence. Paradoxically, this weakened immune response coexists with heightened baseline inflammation, partly due to an increased production of inflammatory mediators by aging immune cells.

- **Gut Microbiota Alterations:** The gut houses trillions of microbes, and changes in this microbiota composition with age can influence immune responses and inflammation.

3. Consequences of Inflammaging:

Chronic inflammation has profound effects on tissue function and is linked to a plethora of age-related diseases:

- **Neurodegenerative Diseases:** Conditions like Alzheimer's and Parkinson's disease are associated with chronic inflammation. In the brain, prolonged inflammation can lead to neuron damage and death.

- **Cardiovascular Diseases:** Chronic inflammation plays a role in atherosclerosis, where inflammatory immune cells contribute to plaque formation in arteries.

- **Metabolic Disorders:** Inflammation is implicated in insulin resistance, a precursor to type 2 diabetes. Fat tissues, especially in obesity, can become inflamed, further exacerbating insulin resistance.

- **Cancer:** Inflammation can promote tumorigenesis by inducing DNA damage, fostering a conducive tumor microenvironment, and facilitating metastasis.

4. Can We Target Inflammaging?

Given its pivotal role in aging and age-related diseases, inflammaging is a prime therapeutic target. Strategies include:

- **Senolytics:** These are drugs that selectively kill senescent cells, potentially reducing the SASP and associated inflammation.

- **Dietary Interventions:** Anti-inflammatory diets, rich in antioxidants and omega-3 fatty acids, can potentially counteract inflammaging.

- **Exercise:** Regular physical activity has anti-inflammatory effects and can mitigate some of the adverse outcomes associated with chronic inflammation.
- **Gut Microbiota Modulation:** Probiotics, prebiotics, and dietary interventions to foster a healthy gut microbiome can potentially reduce systemic inflammation.

Conclusion

Inflammaging, with its pervasive influence on tissue function and disease onset, is a central player in the aging narrative. Recognizing and understanding this chronic inflammatory state offers pathways to mitigate its effects, potentially extending healthspan and delaying the onset of age-related diseases. As research continues to unravel the complexities of inflammaging, it fosters hope that targeting this hallmark could significantly impact the trajectory of human aging.

Molecular Pathways Leading to Inflammaging

Inflammaging, or the persistent low-grade inflammation observed in the elderly, is a significant contributor to various age-related diseases. A better understanding of the molecular pathways leading to inflammaging can offer insights into its origins and provide potential therapeutic targets. Several pathways, intricately interwoven, play a crucial role in the establishment and maintenance of this chronic inflammatory state.

1. NF-κB Signaling:

The nuclear factor-kappa B (NF-κB) pathway is central to inflammation and has been closely linked to the aging process. Under homeostatic conditions, NF-κB remains inactive in the cytoplasm. However, upon exposure to inflammatory stimuli such as cytokines, pathogens, or ROS, the NF-κB pathway becomes activated. This leads to the transcription of genes involved in inflammation, cell adhesion, and immune responses. Chronic activation of NF-κB signaling in aging cells contributes to the persistent production of pro-inflammatory molecules, driving inflammaging.

2. The NLRP3 Inflammasome:

The NLRP3 inflammasome is a multi-protein complex that, once activated, promotes the maturation and secretion of inflammatory cytokines like IL-1β and IL-18. Aging, cellular damage, metabolic imbalances, and mitochondrial dysfunction can all activate the NLRP3 inflammasome, making it a critical player in inflammaging. Moreover, senescent cells exhibit elevated NLRP3 activity, further linking cellular aging and chronic inflammation.

3. JAK-STAT Signaling:

The Janus kinase-signal transducer and activator of transcription (JAK-STAT) pathway plays a role in various cellular processes, including proliferation, differentiation, and immunity. Persistent activation of JAK-STAT signaling in aging tissues, likely due to increased levels of pro-inflammatory cytokines like IL-6, drives chronic inflammation and can contribute to diseases such as atherosclerosis and diabetes.

4. mTOR Pathway:

The mechanistic target of rapamycin (mTOR) pathway regulates cell growth, proliferation, and survival. Overactivity of the mTOR pathway has been observed in aging and is linked to increased production of pro-inflammatory cytokines, thereby promoting inflammaging. Interestingly, inhibition of mTOR, using compounds like rapamycin, has been shown to extend lifespan in various organisms and decrease markers of inflammation.

5. SASP (Senescence-Associated Secretory Phenotype):

Cellular senescence is a state where cells lose their ability to divide but remain metabolically active. One of the defining characteristics of senescent cells is the secretion of SASP, a cocktail of pro-inflammatory cytokines, chemokines, and proteases. This secretory phenotype can induce inflammation in neighboring cells, thereby amplifying the inflammatory response. The accumulation of senescent cells with age contributes significantly to the inflammaging milieu.

6. Gut Microbiome Dysbiosis:

The gut microbiome, a complex ecosystem of microbes residing in our intestines, plays a pivotal role in health and disease. With age, changes in the composition and function of these microbial communities can lead to increased gut permeability and the translocation of bacterial products into circulation. This can activate multiple inflammatory pathways, further exacerbating the chronic inflammatory state.

7. DAMPs and PAMPs:

Damage-associated molecular patterns (DAMPs) and pathogen-associated molecular patterns (PAMPs) are molecules released during cell damage or in response to pathogens, respectively. Recognition of DAMPs and PAMPs by immune cells via pattern recognition receptors, like toll-like receptors (TLRs), can activate inflammatory pathways. With age, the accumulation of DAMPs due to cellular damage and potential dysbiosis-driven PAMPs contribute to heightened inflammatory responses.

Conclusion

Inflammaging is not the result of a single pathway but rather a convergence of multiple molecular mechanisms that become dysregulated with age. By understanding these intricate pathways, researchers aim to identify potential intervention points that could mitigate inflammaging and its deleterious effects, offering a more healthful aging process. The promise lies in leveraging this knowledge to develop therapies that can reduce chronic inflammation and its associated age-related diseases.

Strategies to Modulate Inflammation in Aging

Inflammaging, characterized by chronic, low-grade inflammation, is a significant contributor to the aging process and various age-related diseases. Modulating this inflammatory response can potentially delay aging, extend healthspan, and decrease the risk of age-related pathologies. A myriad of strategies, ranging from lifestyle changes to advanced therapeutic interventions, have emerged over the years to combat inflammaging.

1. Dietary Interventions:

- **Caloric Restriction (CR):** Multiple studies have shown that reducing caloric intake without malnutrition can extend lifespan and healthspan in various organisms. CR reduces levels of pro-inflammatory cytokines and mitigates inflammation, potentially by suppressing NF-κB signaling.
- **Mediterranean Diet:** Rich in fruits, vegetables, olive oil, and fish, the Mediterranean diet is associated with reduced markers of inflammation. Its beneficial effects might be attributed to the high content of antioxidants and anti-inflammatory compounds.
- **Polyphenols:** Found in foods like green tea, berries, and dark chocolate, polyphenols have anti-inflammatory properties and can modulate pathways linked with inflammaging.

2. Physical Activity:

Regular exercise exerts anti-inflammatory effects, reducing cytokine production and enhancing the release of anti-inflammatory myokines from muscles. Exercise also improves metabolic health, reducing the risk of inflammatory metabolic diseases.

3. Sleep and Stress Management:

Chronic stress and sleep deprivation can activate inflammatory pathways. Ensuring adequate sleep and practicing stress-reducing techniques like meditation and deep-breathing exercises can help in lowering inflammation.

4. Pharmacological Interventions:

- **Senolytics:** These are compounds that selectively eliminate senescent cells, which often exhibit the pro-inflammatory senescence-associated secretory phenotype (SASP). By reducing the burden of these cells, senolytics can potentially decrease inflammaging.

- **mTOR Inhibitors:** Drugs like rapamycin, which inhibit the mTOR pathway, have shown promise in reducing inflammation and extending lifespan in preclinical models.
- **Non-Steroidal Anti-Inflammatory Drugs (NSAIDs):** Although commonly used for pain and inflammation, long-term use of NSAIDs as an anti-aging strategy requires careful consideration due to potential side effects.

5. Gut Microbiota Modulation:

- **Probiotics and Prebiotics:** Maintaining a healthy gut microbiota can help in reducing systemic inflammation. Probiotics (beneficial bacteria) and prebiotics (food for these bacteria) can promote a balanced gut environment.
- **Fecal Microbiota Transplantation (FMT):** While still experimental for aging, FMT involves transferring gut microbiota from healthy donors to recipients to restore a balanced microbial community, which could potentially modulate inflammation.

6. Immune System Modulation:

Targeting immune cells, especially overactive or dysregulated components, can help reduce chronic inflammation. Interventions like immune cell depletion or the use of monoclonal antibodies against specific inflammatory mediators are under investigation.

7. Targeted Pathway Inhibition:

Specific inhibitors targeting pathways like NF-κB, JAK-STAT, or the NLRP3 inflammasome can reduce inflammation. However, given the central roles of these pathways in immunity and cell signaling, careful consideration of potential side effects is necessary.

8. Hormonal Therapies:

Hormones like estrogen have anti-inflammatory properties. Hormone replacement therapy, especially in post-menopausal women, might offer benefits in reducing inflammation, though potential risks need to be weighed against benefits.

Conclusion

Combatting inflammaging is a multi-pronged approach that requires a combination of lifestyle modifications and therapeutic interventions. As research advances, we are gaining a clearer picture of the intricacies of inflammaging and the best strategies to modulate it. The hope is that by targeting chronic inflammation, we can pave the way for healthier, more productive aging, reducing the burden of age-related diseases and improving quality of life in our later years.

Chapter 10: Intercellular Communication and the Aging Microenvironment

How Cells Communicate in Tissue Environments

Cells, the fundamental units of life, are not isolated entities; they rely heavily on communication with their neighboring cells to function properly within a multicellular organism. This cellular crosstalk is pivotal for tissue and organ development, homeostasis, and response to environmental changes. In tissue environments, cells employ an array of intricate communication mechanisms to relay and receive messages.

1. Direct Cell-to-Cell Contact:

- **Gap Junctions:** These are protein channels that directly connect neighboring cells, allowing for the exchange of ions, metabolites, and other small molecules. Gap junctions are crucial for processes like cardiac muscle contraction, where synchronization between cells is required.

- **Desmosomes and Adherens Junctions:** While primarily providing structural support by binding cells together, these junctions also facilitate signal transduction pathways that help in cell communication, especially in epithelial and cardiac tissues.

- **Immunological Synapse:** This specialized junction forms between an antigen-presenting cell and a T lymphocyte, enabling the direct transfer of information for immune responses.

2. Paracrine Signaling:

In this mode of communication, cells release signaling molecules into the extracellular fluid, affecting nearby target cells. These signals usually act over short distances.

- **Neurotransmitters:** Neurons communicate at synapses using neurotransmitters. A neuron releases these chemicals, which then bind to receptors on a nearby neuron, eliciting a response.
- **Growth Factors:** These proteins regulate cell growth and differentiation. For instance, fibroblast growth factor (FGF) guides the healing process in wounds by stimulating cell proliferation.

3. Autocrine Signaling:

Here, cells produce signaling molecules that bind to their receptors, effectively allowing cells to signal themselves. This mechanism plays a role in various processes, including tumor cell proliferation, where a cancer cell might release growth factors that stimulate its growth.

4. Endocrine Signaling:

This involves cells releasing hormones into the bloodstream, which can then travel significant distances to act on target cells in distant organs. Examples include insulin, which regulates glucose uptake in cells, and thyroid hormones, which influence metabolism.

5. Juxtacrine Signaling:

In juxtacrine signaling, a cell presents a signal on its surface, which interacts with receptors on a neighboring cell, inducing a change. This type of communication is evident in the Delta-Notch signaling pathway, crucial for differentiation and tissue development.

6. Extracellular Vesicles:

Recent research has unveiled the significance of extracellular vesicles, such as exosomes, in cell communication. Cells release these vesicles containing proteins, lipids, and nucleic acids into the extracellular space, which can then be taken up by neighboring or distant cells, modulating their function.

7. Matrix Signaling:

The extracellular matrix (ECM) is not just a structural scaffold but also plays an active role in cellular signaling. Cells interact with and receive signals from the ECM components through integrins and other receptors. This interaction influences cell migration, differentiation, and survival.

8. Mechanical Signaling:

Physical forces, such as those from fluid flow or tissue stretching, can be sensed by cells and converted into biochemical signals. For instance, endothelial cells lining blood vessels can detect changes in blood flow and adjust their function accordingly.

Conclusion

Cellular communication in tissue environments is a beautifully orchestrated process, ensuring the harmonious functioning of the organism. The modes of communication are diverse, and their interplay is central to development, tissue repair, immune responses, and many other physiological processes. Disruptions in these communication pathways can lead to diseases like cancer, autoimmune disorders, and degenerative diseases. Understanding these intricate signaling pathways is not only essential for basic biology but also holds the key to novel therapeutic interventions for various ailments.

Changes in Intercellular Communication with Age

The intricate dance of cellular communication is fundamental to the harmonious operation of multicellular organisms. From development and growth to maintenance and repair, cells rely on signals from their neighbors to make decisions. However, as organisms age, there are profound changes in the way cells communicate with each other. These alterations can influence tissue function, drive age-related pathologies, and impact the overall health and longevity of an organism.

1. Gap Junctional Communication:

Gap junctions, the direct conduits for intercellular exchange of ions and small molecules, display reduced efficiency with age. The age-related decline in gap junctional communication can disrupt tissue synchronization. For instance, in cardiac tissues, this can potentially lead to arrhythmias.

2. Changes in Paracrine Signaling:

Growth factors, cytokines, and other signaling molecules released by cells to act on nearby cells can change with age. An example is the age-related decline in the production of certain growth factors that promote neuronal survival and differentiation, contributing to neural degeneration. Conversely, there's an increase in pro-inflammatory cytokines, such as interleukin-6 (IL-6) and tumor necrosis factor-alpha (TNF-α), promoting a state of chronic low-grade inflammation termed "inflammaging."

3. Altered Autocrine Feedback Loops:

Aging can alter autocrine signals, where cells signal themselves. An example is seen in immune cells. With age, some immune cells exhibit increased autocrine production of inflammatory molecules, further exacerbating the inflammaging state.

4. Endocrine Disruptions:

With advancing age, there's a marked change in the production, release, and action of various hormones. Reduced insulin sensitivity in peripheral tissues, decline in growth hormone and sex steroid levels, and altered circadian release of melatonin are just a few examples. These endocrine shifts can affect metabolism, sleep, mood, and overall vitality.

5. Disruptions in Juxtacrine Signaling:

The direct interactions between adjacent cells, critical for processes like differentiation, can be affected by age. For instance, stem cell niches rely on juxtacrine signals from supporting cells to maintain stemness. Aging can disrupt these signals, leading to reduced stem cell function and compromised tissue repair.

6. Extracellular Vesicle Communication:

Recent studies suggest that the content and release of extracellular vesicles, like exosomes, change with age. These vesicles can carry proteins, lipids, and nucleic acids. Age-related modifications in vesicle content can influence processes like angiogenesis, immune responses, and inter-organ communication.

7. Extracellular Matrix and Integrin Signaling:

The extracellular matrix (ECM) undergoes significant structural and compositional changes with age. These changes can affect integrin-mediated signals that cells receive from the ECM, influencing cell migration, survival, and differentiation. For instance, stiffening of the ECM with age can drive fibrosis and disrupt tissue function.

8. Mechanical Signaling Changes:

Aging tissues often experience changes in mechanical properties, such as increased stiffness. Cells can sense these mechanical changes and convert them into biochemical signals. In aged tissues, altered mechanical signaling can promote pathological states like fibrosis, inflammation, and impaired regenerative capacity.

Conclusion

Intercellular communication networks are dynamic and can change profoundly with age. These changes are not just passive consequences of aging but can actively drive the aging process. From the subdued whispers of gap junctions to the loud cries of inflammaging, age-related disruptions in cellular communication impact every corner of an organism's biology. Understanding these changes holds promise for developing interventions that can improve healthspan, combat age-associated pathologies, and perhaps even rejuvenate tissues. As we peel back the layers of the aging process, the significance of intercellular communication stands out as a central theme and a potential therapeutic target.

The Aged Microenvironment and Its Influence on Cell Behavior

Every cell in our body exists within a specialized microenvironment, an intricate web of neighboring cells, extracellular matrix (ECM), signaling molecules, and mechanical cues. This microenvironment, or niche, plays a critical role in determining the fate, function, and behavior of a cell. As organisms age, the microenvironment undergoes significant changes, often referred to as the "aged microenvironment," which in turn influences cell behavior in multiple ways.

1. Structural and Compositional Changes in the ECM:

One of the most conspicuous changes in the aged microenvironment is the alteration in the ECM. The ECM provides mechanical support and relays biochemical cues to cells. With age, there's an increase in matrix stiffness, a buildup of cross-linked collagen, and a decline in elastin, making tissues less elastic and more fibrotic. These changes can affect cell behavior by altering their adherence, migration, and signaling pathways. For instance, a stiffer matrix can promote a more invasive behavior in cancer cells.

2. Altered Signaling Molecule Profiles:

The aged microenvironment often has altered levels of signaling molecules, like growth factors and cytokines. For example, there's a notable increase in pro-inflammatory molecules, such as IL-6 and TNF-α, in aged tissues. This shift can drive chronic inflammation, influencing cellular behaviors like proliferation, differentiation, and immune response. Chronic inflammation can also exacerbate age-related diseases, including atherosclerosis and neurodegenerative conditions.

3. Oxidative Stress:

Aging tissues often experience higher levels of reactive oxygen species (ROS) due to mitochondrial dysfunction and other factors. Elevated ROS can damage cellular components and alter the behavior of cells in the microenvironment. For instance, oxidative stress can induce

DNA damage, alter cell signaling pathways, and even trigger cellular senescence.

4. Senescent Cells and the SASP:

One of the hallmarks of the aged microenvironment is the accumulation of senescent cells – cells that have ceased to divide but remain metabolically active. These cells release a plethora of molecules, known as the senescence-associated secretory phenotype (SASP), which includes inflammatory cytokines, growth factors, and proteases. The SASP can modulate the behavior of neighboring cells, often in detrimental ways. For instance, the SASP can promote inflammation, suppress stem cell function, and even drive cancer progression.

5. Decline in Stem Cell Niche Function:

Stem cells reside in specialized niches that maintain their quiescence, self-renewal, and differentiation potential. The aged microenvironment often compromises these niches. Altered ECM, reduced levels of supportive growth factors, and increased inflammatory signals can affect stem cell behavior, leading to reduced regenerative capacity in aged tissues.

6. Vascular Changes:

Aged tissues often exhibit altered vasculature, with reduced capillary density and compromised endothelial function. This can affect the delivery of nutrients and oxygen, impacting cell metabolism and function. Moreover, endothelial cells in aged tissues might release altered sets of signaling molecules, influencing cell behavior in the vicinity.

Conclusion

The microenvironment is like the soil in which cells thrive, and just as the quality of soil affects plant health, the characteristics of the microenvironment influence cell behavior. The aged microenvironment, with its myriad changes, can push cells towards behaviors that are often associated with age-related pathologies. Understanding these alterations and their impact on cells is not only pivotal for the basic understanding of aging but also offers insights into therapeutic avenues.

By rejuvenating the aged microenvironment or shielding cells from its detrimental cues, it might be possible to ameliorate age-related diseases and possibly extend healthspan.

Chapter 11: Hallmarks of Aging

An Integrated View of the Major Cellular and Molecular Changes During Aging

Aging is an intricate and multifaceted process, manifesting through a cascade of cellular and molecular changes. While each change might appear as an isolated event, they are deeply interwoven, contributing to a collective orchestra that dictates the aging rhythm of an organism. To truly understand aging, one must view these changes not as individual strings but as parts of an interconnected web.

1. DNA Damage and Repair Pathways:

At the molecular level, one of the primary changes observed with aging is the accumulation of DNA damage. Environmental stressors, metabolic by-products, and replication errors can induce mutations. While cells have evolved repair mechanisms to rectify these damages, their efficiency wanes with age. Persistent DNA damage can activate pathways leading to apoptosis or senescence, impacting tissue homeostasis.

2. Telomere Shortening:

Telomeres, the protective caps of chromosomes, shorten with each cell division. Aging cells often exhibit critically short telomeres, which can cause genomic instability and cell cycle arrest. Telomerase, an enzyme that extends telomeres, has therapeutic potential, but its unregulated activity could also lead to malignancies.

3. Mitochondrial Dysfunction:

Mitochondria, the powerhouses of the cell, show a decline in their function with age. They produce more reactive oxygen species (ROS) and less ATP, leading to energy depletion and oxidative stress. These perturbations can influence various cellular processes, from metabolism to cell death.

4. Protein Misfolding and Aggregation:

Aging cells often struggle with maintaining protein quality. There's an accumulation of misfolded or aggregated proteins, as processes like autophagy and proteasomal degradation become less efficient. Such protein aggregates can be toxic and are characteristic of several age-related diseases, including Alzheimer's and Parkinson's.

5. Epigenetic Alterations:

The epigenome, which influences gene expression without altering the DNA sequence, undergoes significant changes during aging. Histone modifications, DNA methylation patterns, and non-coding RNA profiles evolve, affecting the cellular transcriptome and thereby influencing cell behavior and function.

6. Cellular Senescence and SASP:

A hallmark of aging is the accumulation of senescent cells, which cease to divide but remain metabolically active. These cells release a myriad of factors, the senescence-associated secretory phenotype (SASP), which can modulate the microenvironment, often promoting inflammation and tissue dysfunction.

7. Inflammation and Immune Dysfunction:

Chronic low-grade inflammation, or "inflammaging," is a consistent feature of aged organisms. This is coupled with immune senescence, where the immune system's efficiency to combat infections and clear dysfunctional cells diminishes. The combined effect not only increases vulnerability to diseases but also promotes various age-related pathologies.

8. Altered Intercellular Communication:

The signaling pathways and molecules that cells use to communicate undergo changes with age. This affects tissue synchronization, hormonal balance, and the responsiveness of cells to their environment. Miscommunication can lead to pathologies like insulin resistance or disrupted circadian rhythms.

9. Stem Cell Exhaustion:

Stem cells, vital for tissue repair and regeneration, lose their potency with age. Their niches become less supportive, and their intrinsic capacity to differentiate and proliferate diminishes, leading to reduced regenerative potential in aged tissues.

Conclusion

Aging is like a symphony, with each cellular and molecular change contributing a unique note. While these changes may begin as isolated events, they eventually intertwine, influencing, and exacerbating each other. It's this integrated view of aging that holds the promise of comprehensive therapeutic strategies. By understanding how these mechanisms intersect and amplify the aging process, scientists are better poised to intervene, modulate, or even reverse some of these pathways, paving the way for healthier aging.

Synthesis of Earlier Chapters and the Interplay Between Different Biological Processes

Throughout this exploration of the biology of aging, we've journeyed across various cellular and molecular landscapes, from the intricacies of DNA to the complexities of cellular communication. While each chapter has provided an in-depth analysis of a specific component, it's essential to synthesize these insights and understand the interplay among the various biological processes. Aging is not a result of isolated events but is rather a cumulative outcome of interconnected phenomena.

1. DNA, Telomeres, and Cellular Health:

At the heart of cellular biology lies DNA. As explored in earlier chapters, DNA sustains damage over time, and while repair pathways work diligently to rectify errors, their efficiency declines with age. Parallelly, the shortening of telomeres–protective caps on chromosomes–acts as a molecular clock, with each division bringing the cell closer to its eventual senescence. Both these processes, if unchecked, lead to cellular dysfunction, either through mutations that can cause diseases or via cellular senescence that disrupts tissue function.

2. The Mitochondrial Connection:

Mitochondrial dysfunction, characterized by diminished energy production and increased ROS, is intrinsically linked to DNA damage. ROS can cause oxidative stress, damaging DNA, proteins, and lipids. Moreover, mitochondrial DNA, which lacks the protective histones of nuclear DNA, is particularly vulnerable. This interplay between mitochondrial dysfunction and genomic instability is a vicious cycle, each exacerbating the other.

3. Proteostasis, Cellular Senescence, and the Tissue Microenvironment:

Protein quality control, vital for cellular health, diminishes with age, leading to protein misfolding and aggregation. This decline can activate stress responses that push cells into senescence. Senescent cells, in turn, secrete a plethora of molecules (SASP) that can affect the microenvironment. These molecules can induce inflammation, alter ECM properties, and even influence neighboring cells' behavior, leading to tissue dysfunction.

4. Epigenetics, Cellular Behavior, and Communication:

Epigenetic changes alter gene expression patterns, thereby influencing cellular behavior and fate. This epigenetic landscape evolves with age, shaped by both intrinsic and extrinsic factors. These changes in gene expression can alter cellular communication patterns, affecting hormonal signaling, growth factor release, and more. In turn, altered intercellular communication can feedback and shape the epigenetic landscape, highlighting the intricate dance between these two realms.

5. Inflammation, Immune Dysfunction, and Systemic Aging:

Inflammaging, the chronic low-grade inflammation observed in aged organisms, can arise from various sources: senescent cells releasing pro-inflammatory SASP, mitochondrial dysfunction leading to ROS production, or DNA damage activating inflammatory pathways. Concurrently, the aging immune system becomes less efficient in clearing pathogens and dysfunctional cells. This combined state of heightened inflammation and reduced immune competence accelerates tissue aging and increases vulnerability to diseases.

6. The Stem Cell, Niche, and Regeneration Interplay:

Aging is not just about decline but also about reduced capacity for renewal. Stem cells, our reservoir for tissue regeneration, decline in function with age. Their niches, influenced by the aged microenvironment, become less supportive. Furthermore, factors like DNA damage, telomere shortening, and inflammaging can directly impact stem cell potency.

Conclusion

In this synthesis, it becomes evident that the biology of aging is a tapestry of intertwined threads. Each biological process, while having its unique trajectory, is deeply connected to others. Interventions in one realm can ripple across others, amplifying or mitigating aging effects. This interconnectedness provides both challenges and opportunities. While it means that disruptions can have systemic effects, it also implies that targeted interventions can have widespread benefits. By understanding the interplay between different biological processes, we move closer to holistic strategies that can address aging in its multifaceted glory.

Chapter 12: Interventions and the Future of Age Biology

Current and Potential Interventions at Cellular and Molecular Levels

Aging, while a natural process, has been the subject of extensive scientific scrutiny, especially with the increasing understanding of its underlying cellular and molecular mechanisms. As these mechanisms have come to light, researchers have also begun to develop a myriad of interventions aiming to mitigate, reverse, or delay the adverse effects of aging. This chapter delves into some of the most promising current and potential interventions at the cellular and molecular levels.

1. Telomerase Activation:

Given the critical role of telomere shortening in cellular senescence and aging, one avenue of intervention is the activation of telomerase. This enzyme can add DNA sequences to the ends of chromosomes, effectively extending telomeres. While initial studies have shown promise in extending cell lifespan in vitro, potential risks, like the unintended promotion of cancer, require thorough investigation.

2. Senolytics:

Senolytics are a class of drugs designed to selectively eliminate senescent cells from tissues. By reducing the number of these dysfunctional cells and their associated secretory phenotype (SASP), researchers aim to rejuvenate tissues and reduce age-related inflammation. Initial trials in mice have shown positive results, with enhanced healthspan and reduced evidence of age-associated pathologies.

3. Mitochondrial Therapies:

Given the central role of mitochondria in energy production and their association with aging, strategies to enhance mitochondrial function are of significant interest. This includes antioxidants that can neutralize reactive oxygen species (ROS) and compounds that can stimulate mitochondrial biogenesis.

4. Protein Homeostasis Modulators:

With age, the protein quality control mechanisms, like autophagy and the ubiquitin-proteasome system, become less efficient. Enhancing these pathways can reduce the accumulation of misfolded proteins. Caloric restriction and certain compounds, like rapamycin, have shown promise in this regard.

5. Epigenetic Rejuvenation:

As we've learned, epigenetic changes accumulate with age, altering gene expression patterns. Techniques that can reset the epigenome to a more "youthful" state are being explored. Recent breakthroughs in cellular reprogramming, where mature cells can be reverted to stem-like states, offer glimpses into potential epigenetic rejuvenation strategies.

6. Dietary and Metabolic Interventions:

Dietary interventions, like caloric restriction (CR) and intermittent fasting, have shown robust anti-aging effects across various species. These interventions affect a plethora of cellular and molecular pathways, from enhancing autophagy to modulating energy-sensing pathways like mTOR and AMPK. Mimetics of CR, such as resveratrol and metformin, are also under investigation for their potential anti-aging benefits.

7. Stem Cell Therapies:

Stem cells have the potential to replace or regenerate tissues that have deteriorated with age. Interventions ranging from the transplantation of exogenous stem cells to the rejuvenation of endogenous stem cell populations are being explored. While still in its early days, the promise of restoring tissue function through stem cells is tantalizing.

8. Modulating Intercellular Communication:

Given the importance of cellular communication in tissue homeostasis, interventions aim to restore or enhance these signaling pathways. This includes modulating hormonal signaling, enhancing growth
factor responses, or inhibiting detrimental signaling cascades associated with aging.

Conclusion

As our understanding of the cellular and molecular underpinnings
of aging deepens, the toolbox of interventions continues to expand.
These approaches, often interrelated, offer the potential not only to
extend lifespan but, more importantly, to enhance healthspan – the
period of life spent in good health. While many of these interventions
are in early stages, with rigorous research and careful application, they
represent the frontier of a future where aging might be addressed at
its very roots.

Promising Research Directions and Therapeutic Strategies

The pursuit of understanding aging has never been more vigorous. As
we have unraveled some of the core mysteries of the aging process at
the cellular and molecular levels, we've concurrently ignited a surge in
research aimed at therapeutic strategies. While the previous sections
delved into current interventions, this section will illuminate the horizon, exploring emerging research directions and therapies that could
redefine our approach to aging.

1. Genomic Editing and CRISPR Technology:

One of the most transformative discoveries in recent biology is
CRISPR-Cas9, a genome-editing tool. This technology allows scientists
to "edit" sequences within the genome with unprecedented precision.
For aging research, CRISPR could be used to correct mutations that
accumulate over time, introduce protective genes, or even modulate
the expression of genes linked with longevity. Ongoing research is

exploring the potential benefits and ethical considerations of such interventions.

2. Extracellular Vesicles (EVs) and Cell-to-Cell Communication:

Recent discoveries highlight the importance of EVs, tiny vesicles released by cells, in intercellular communication. These vesicles carry proteins, lipids, and nucleic acids, influencing the behavior of recipient cells. In the context of aging, understanding and modulating EV-mediated communication could pave the way for interventions that rejuvenate tissues or mitigate age-related decline.

3. Advanced Immunotherapies:

The immune system's decline with age, termed immunosenescence, plays a pivotal role in susceptibility to diseases and chronic inflammation. Novel immunotherapies, which harness or modulate the immune system, hold promise. For instance, chimeric antigen receptor (CAR) T-cell therapies, which supercharge the immune system to target specific cells, might be repurposed to address aging-related challenges, like clearing senescent cells.

4. Synthetic Biology and Designing Longevity:

Synthetic biology involves designing and constructing new biological entities or redesigning existing ones. For aging, this could mean creating synthetic organisms or pathways that counteract age-related deterioration. Imagine microbes engineered to bolster gut health in the elderly or synthetic pathways that amplify cellular repair mechanisms.

5. Artificial Intelligence and Multi-Omics Data Analysis:

Aging is multifaceted, and its study produces vast, complex datasets. Employing artificial intelligence (AI) and machine learning to analyze genomic, proteomic, metabolomic, and other 'omics' data can reveal patterns and insights previously inaccessible. These insights might point to novel drug targets, predictive biomarkers of aging, or individualized therapeutic strategies.

6. Gut Microbiome and Aging:

Emerging evidence underscores the intimate relationship between the gut microbiome's composition and healthspan. Age-related shifts in microbiome diversity can influence inflammation, metabolism, and even neurological health. Interventions that restore or optimize the gut microbiota, like precision probiotics or fecal transplants, are gaining traction as potential anti-aging strategies.

7. Bioinformatics and Drug Repurposing:

Many existing drugs, approved for other conditions, might have hitherto unrecognized anti-aging properties. Using bioinformatics to sift through vast drug databases, researchers can identify candidates for repurposing. For instance, metformin, a diabetes drug, is now under investigation for its potential lifespan-extending properties.

8. Systems Biology and Holistic Approaches:

Rather than focusing on isolated pathways, a systems biology approach considers the organism as an intricate, interconnected network. By modeling these networks, researchers can identify crucial nodes and interventions that have system-wide impacts, providing a holistic approach to tackling aging.

Conclusion

The horizon of aging research is dazzlingly bright. With every emerging technology and innovative approach, we inch closer to a world where aging's detrimental effects are mitigated, if not reversed. While challenges abound, the confluence of biology, technology, and ingenuity promises a future where aging is not a decline but a new chapter of continued vitality.

Ethical Considerations and the Future of Anti-Aging Interventions

The pursuit of extending human lifespan, while an ancient dream, is now more palpable than ever due to the rapid advancements in biotechnology and our understanding of the aging process. However, as with all profound shifts in our capabilities, there are profound ethical considerations that society must grapple with. The potential for anti-aging interventions does not just reshape our biology but raises philosophical, societal, and moral dilemmas about the nature of human existence.

1. Equity and Access:

One of the foremost concerns is the equitable access to these potential anti-aging treatments. There's a genuine risk that such interventions, particularly in their early stages, will be expensive and available only to the wealthy. This could exacerbate existing social inequalities, where the affluent not only have more resources but also live significantly longer, healthier lives than the less fortunate.

2. Overpopulation and Resource Strain:

If humans can significantly extend their lifespans, the resultant population growth could strain Earth's already limited resources. Food, water, housing, and energy demands could skyrocket, leading to intensified competition, potential conflicts, and environmental degradation. Additionally, increased longevity without improved healthspan could lead to a surge in the elderly population requiring extensive care.

3. Cultural and Generational Dynamics:

Longer lifespans will reshape societal structures and dynamics. Traditionally, societies have relied on generational turnover to infuse new ideas and perspectives. But if several generations coexist for extended periods, it could affect everything from job markets (with older individuals occupying positions for longer) to cultural shifts (which might slow if older generations, with established beliefs, dominate societal discourse).

4. Personal Identity and the Nature of Life:

From a philosophical perspective, what does it mean for our identity if we can live for significantly extended periods? Part of the human experience has always been the recognition of our own mortality. If

that changes, how do we perceive time, life's purpose, and our re-
lationships? Life stages, such as childhood, adulthood, and old age,
would require redefinition.

5. Medical and Biological Risks:

Every intervention carries risks. While the intent of anti-aging treatments is to promote health, there's always the possibility of unforeseen
side effects, especially when modifying complex systems like human
biology. For instance, while activating telomerase might extend cellular life, it also has potential implications for increased cancer risks.

6. Defining "Natural":

There's a philosophical debate over what is deemed 'natural'. If
aging is a natural process, is halting or reversing it an affront to the
natural order of things? Or, conversely, is it a natural progression of
human evolution to use technology and knowledge to enhance our
own biology?

7. Economic Implications:

A society with a large proportion of long-living individuals will need
to reconsider economic models. Retirement ages, pension systems,
healthcare funding, and even concepts like inheritance could all face
disruption and require rethinking.

Conclusion

While the scientific endeavor to understand and potentially combat
aging is commendable, it does not exist in a vacuum. Society, as a
collective, needs to engage in a robust dialogue about the implications
of such profound changes. Ethical considerations, in many ways, are
as intricate and complex as the biological challenges of aging. The
future of anti-aging interventions is not just a journey of biology but a
deep reflection on the values, principles, and structures that underpin
human civilization. As we tread this path, it's imperative to do so with
foresight, empathy, and a profound respect for the interconnectedness
of life.

Definitions of Key Terms and Concepts

1. **Aging**: A biological process characterized by a decline in an organism's ability to maintain homeostasis, leading to decreased functional capabilities and increased vulnerability to diseases and death.

2. **Autophagy**: A cellular process responsible for the degradation and recycling of cytoplasmic components, which may include dysfunctional cellular organelles or aggregated proteins.

3. **Bioinformatics**: The application of statistical and computational tools to the field of biology, especially used in analyzing and integrating vast amounts of biological data.

4. **Cell Cycle**: A sequence of events by which a cell duplicates its content and divides into two.

5. **Cellular Senescence**: The phenomenon where a cell loses its ability to divide and grow. Though senescent cells remain alive and metabolically active, they can have altered functions that might contribute to aging and various diseases.

6. **Chronological Age**: The actual age of an organism or individual based on time elapsed since birth.

7. **CRISPR-Cas9**: A revolutionary gene-editing technique that can target specific sequences within the genome, offering potential therapies for genetic disorders.

8. **DNA Damage**: Anomalies and alterations in the normal structure of DNA, which could result from exposure to mutagens or mistakes in DNA replication.

9. **Epigenetics**: The study of heritable changes in gene function that do not involve changes in the DNA sequence itself, such as DNA methylation and histone modification.

10. **Extracellular Vesicles (EVs)**: Tiny membrane-bound particles released from cells, known to play roles in cell-to-cell communication, and might also be involved in various pathological conditions.

11. **Genomic Editing**: Techniques used to make precise changes in the genes of organisms, including adding, removing, or replacing DNA.

12. **Immunosenescence**: The decline in the efficiency of the immune system as a result of aging.

13. **Inflammaging**: Chronic, low-grade inflammation observed as a common symptom of aging, contributing to age-associated morbidity and mortality.

14. **Intercellular Communication**: Mechanisms by which cells exchange information with each other, ensuring coordination and proper function at the tissue or organism level.

15. **Mitochondria**: Cell organelles primarily responsible for generating energy in the form of ATP. Often referred to as the "powerhouse" of the cell.

16. **Mitochondrial Dysfunction**: Impairment in the normal functioning of mitochondria, contributing to a variety of cellular problems and diseases.

17. **Proteostasis**: A cellular process that ensures the stability, folding, and proper function of proteins within the cell.

18. **Reactive Oxygen Species (ROS)**: Molecules containing oxygen that can react easily with other molecules in a cell, potentially causing damage. They are a natural byproduct of the normal metabolism of oxygen and play roles in cell signaling and homeostasis.

19. **Signaling Pathways**: A cascade of molecular events within a cell that leads to a specific response. This series of reactions is initiated when a molecule, such as a hormone or neurotransmitter, binds to a receptor on the cell membrane.

20. **Stem Cells**: Unique cells with the potential to differentiate into any cell type in the body and play critical roles in repair, regeneration, and maintenance of tissue.

21. **Telomerase**: An enzyme responsible for maintaining the length of telomeres, offering potential protective effects against cellular aging.

22. **Telomeres**: Protective caps at the ends of chromosomes that shorten as cells divide. Their length can serve as a potential marker of cellular age and overall health.

23. **Therapeutic Interventions**: Procedures or treatments applied to modify, alleviate, or prevent a specific health condition or improve overall health.

24. **Tissue Aging**: Changes at the tissue level, often marked by reduced regenerative potential and function, contributing to the organism's aging process.

25. **Tissue Environment**: The specific conditions, signals, and structures in a localized area within an organism where cells reside and function.

26. **Biological Age**: An assessment of an organism's health and physiological condition relative to its chronological age, often considered a more relevant predictor of health, longevity, and vulnerability to diseases.

27. **DNA Repair Pathways**: Cellular mechanisms activated in response to DNA damage, aiming to maintain genomic integrity.

28. **Protein Quality Control**: Cellular processes ensuring that proteins achieve and maintain their correct 3D structures and ensuring the degradation of misfolded or damaged proteins.